RESTORATIVE YOGA

ESSENTIAL POSES FOR RELAXATION, BALANCED CHAKRA ENERGIES AND HEALING

TABLE OF CONTENTS

INTRODUCTION

Restorative yoga is an exercise that revolves around slowing down and opening the body through passive stretching. If you're in a therapeutic class, you can barely move, with just a few posts over an hour. It is a very different experience from most contemporary yoga. Most yoga classes are an active exercise in which you move from pose to pose, build heat, and increase your strength and flexibility equally. The general trend in yoga is more athletic and acrobatic practice styles. During long restorative yoga periods, your muscles can relax deeply. It is a unique feeling because the accessories, instead of your flesh, are used to support your body. Restorative classes are very gentle, making them an excellent addition to increasingly dynamic practices (just as our bustling lives) and a great counteractant to stretch. Silence is a powerful exercise.

Clinical research on restorative yoga has shown that it can reduce depression in cancer survivors; improve symptoms of anxiety, depression, and pain in cancer patients; and help patients control the toxicity of cancer treatments. Restorative yoga is a safe, gentle, and gentle practice that can help you learn to relax and recharge. You also cultivate the essential skills of self-awareness. More and more research is published on the benefits of 'stress reduction' techniques such as yoga and meditation. Taking time to break free from the tension, breathe, and focus your attention can be a welcome (and sometimes rare) break from the faster pace of modern life.

A central theme of yoga is to experience a balance between effort and ease. In restorative yoga, we balance the luxury of living in silence and relaxation with sustained, lively, and focused attention. These two components cooperate to make a pleasant and engaging experience. Typically, a therapeutic class focuses on spending long periods relaxing and breathing relaxing yoga poses, although an exercise may include some gentle movements. Restorative yoga is safe and accessible to more people due to the use of 'accessories' to support the postures. You can use blankets, pillows (large pillows), blocks, and straps to effortlessly sit in different poses. (More on accessories in a moment).

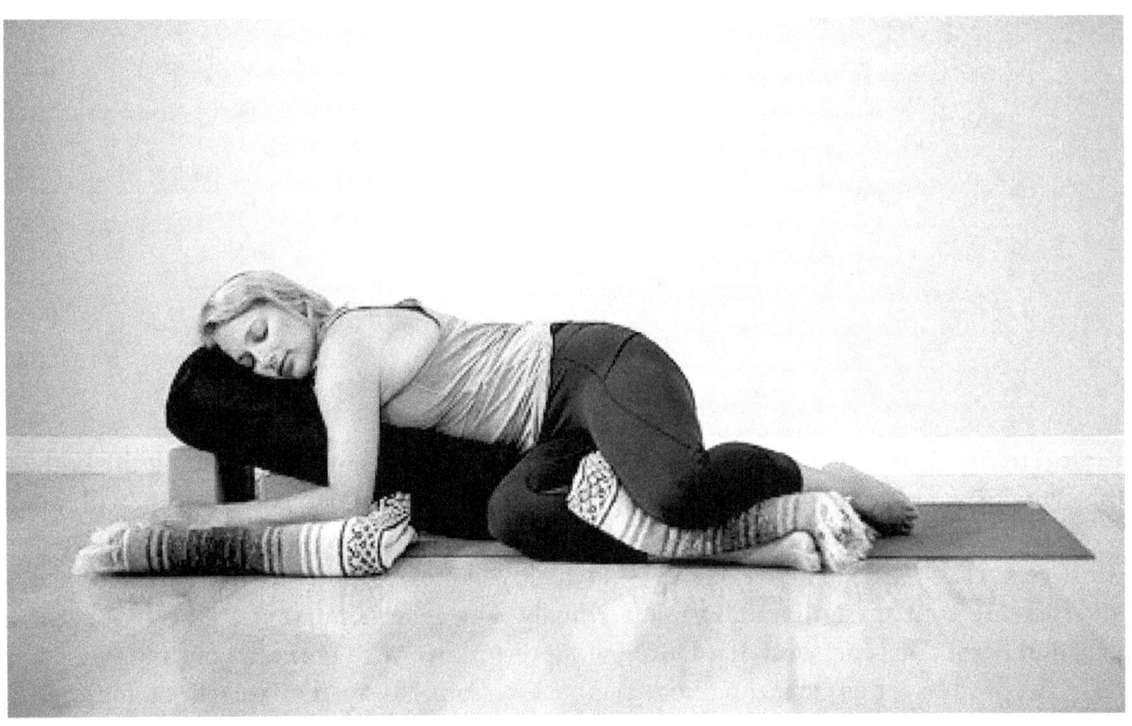

Some general guidelines are:

•	Although most of these poses are gentle, if you have physical concerns, talk to your doctor about integrating yoga into your lifestyle.

•	Give yourself enough time in the pose to feel good. Get comfortable so you can rest in any position for at least five minutes, longer if you feel good.

•	Also, take the time to get out of the poses. Don't rush to move or stand up again. Be present for the different feelings of silence and smooth movements.

•	Keep it simple. As you relax, you will notice your attention drift. Stay relaxed and breathe, again focusing your attention on the feeling of letting go and the subtle movements of your breathing.

I am happy to share my restorative practice with you. Every week I see how this gentle practice can change a person's feelings, not only physically, but also at the level of the intellect, emotion, psyche/mind.

Śavāsana, or corpse pose, may be familiar to you if you have taken yoga classes in a studio or gym. This 'last relaxation pose' generally lasts for five to fifteen minutes and means that you rest on your back, consciously relax the tension and strain on yourself, and breathe gently. I always start and end my recovery lesson with this pose.

It is the simple and unadorned experience of paying attention to yourself over some time, noticing how you feel the tension and how much you can release it. I encourage you to spend at least ten minutes in śavāsana. Give yourself time to feel relaxed and focused on your breathing. Be patient and just enjoy being with yourself, realizing it.

It takes a long time to get out of the pose: remember how much time and care you spend going into softness and silence. Keep those properties smooth, even as you begin to move slowly, starting with your fingers and toes and gradually spreading the movements to all the joints, to yourself. Be there and enjoy the feeling of 'bringing life' back to your bones and muscles. Surround yourself by your side and enjoy some relaxed breaths before slowly rolling up to spend some time sitting. Practicing yoga can be like having a conversation with yourself: noticing, answering, asking questions, learning. I hope we can start our discussion, using these videos and their experiences for dialogue.

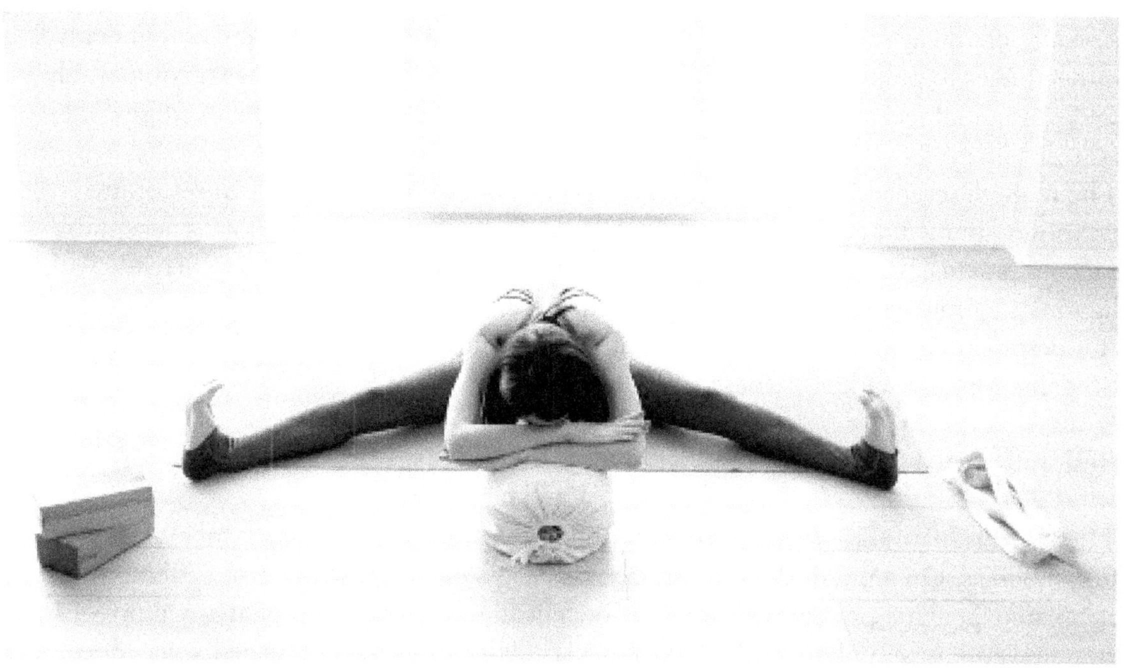

What is restorative yoga?

Restorative yoga is a feeding type of yoga that extends profoundly, latently, and holds fewer postures for more extended periods. Unlike some of the more active or "yang" types of yoga, restorative yoga encourages us to slow down, let go, and suspend activities, both physical and mental. By doing this, it is an exercise that relaxes the body and mind, bridging the gap between the two. Restorative classes use accessories to promote maximum comfort, as students are invited to melt deeply into each pose.

Judith Hanson Lasater made the practice prevalent in the United States in the 1970s. Her training and offering grew out of the teachings of the famous B.K.S. "We work very hard in our lives and, although we can sleep, we seldom set aside the effort to unwind. Remedial yoga presents assist us in figuring out how to rest profoundly and totally. By intentionally bringing a feeling of harmony and serenity to the body, restorative yoga helps us discover our innate ability to be comfortable with the present moment. There is no other primary purpose in restorative yoga that is relaxing, real, and complete.

Restorative yoga versus yin yoga

Restorative yoga and yin yoga are frequently befuddled. While there are numerous likenesses between the two, they are not indistinguishable practices. The two structures convey "yin" vitality, which implies they are moderate activities that work to discharge pressure put away somewhere down in the body. Both are inactive practices that control understudies to plunge profound into presents. Thus, they regularly have a comparable and substantial feel and impact on understudies toward the finish of the exercise.

The main differences are reduced to the level of comfort and purpose. In restorative yoga, the poses are meant to be completely comfortable, while some discomfort is acceptable in a yin practice. Restorative postures focus on rest, while yin yoga works correctly with ligaments, joints, fascial tissue, and bones.
But despite their differences, inner balance and silence are common to both practices. Students who love either of these often love the other.

Restorative yoga benefits

The benefits of restorative yoga are comprehensive and reach physical, mental, and emotional bodies. On a physical level, this exercise helps balance the nervous system, improve sleep, and facilitate physical healing. It is beneficial for the recovery of many types of injuries; however, it is fundamental to counsel a **specialist or an accomplished yoga educator** before working out, in case there are contraindications between a pose and your condition.

At the psychological and passionate level, therapeutic yoga helps quiet the brain, lessen pressure, and direct feelings. One of the ways it this by activating the parasympathetic nervous system, also known as our "digestive and rest system." As we deepen our breathing, we inhale deeper into the abdomen, and as we sink deeper into each posture, we initiate the relaxation response, triggering the parasympathetic nervous system. This decreases the production of stress hormones, allowing both the body and the mind to know that you can rest comfortably.

Restorative yoga is an escape from the chaos of everyday life. It promotes general well-being by providing the ability to distance yourself from anything that captures it is a demonstration of self-esteem that reestablishes the body to various levels, discharging and rebalancing our vitality supplies.

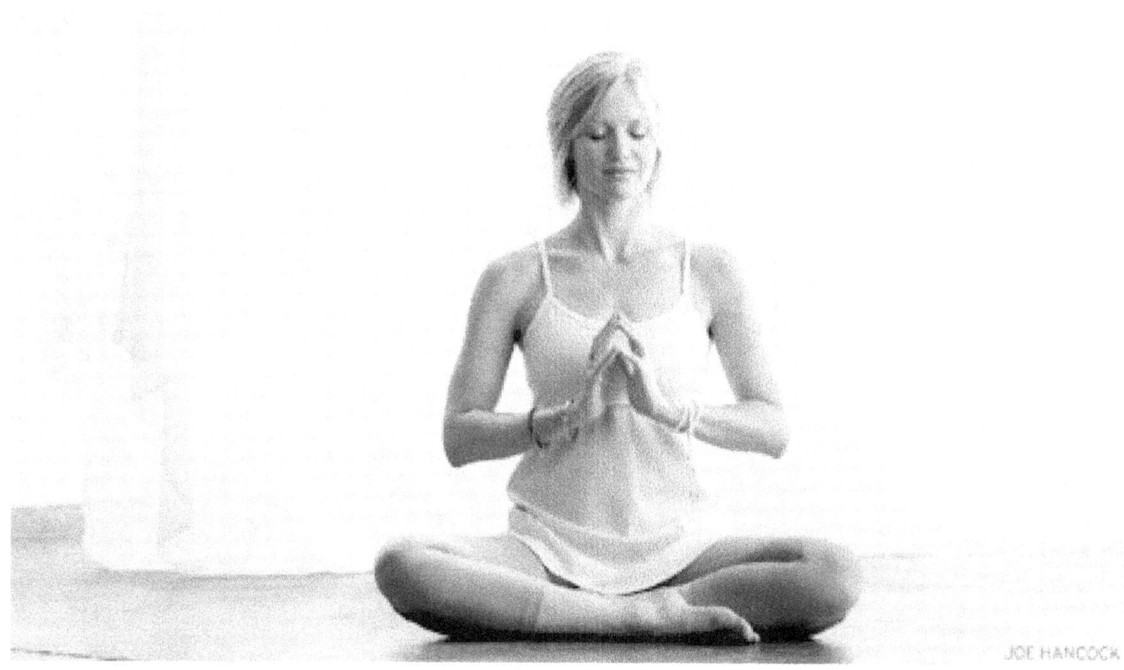

CLEAR AND BALANCE CHAKRA ENERGIES

Everything in our universe emanates vitality, from the huge mountain or sea to the littlest piece of sod to every cell in our body. The entirety of our cells produces vitality in various manners, and multiple cells will emit multiple kinds of intensity, relying upon where they are in the body and what their activity is.

 should come as no surprise, given the specialized nature of your body's energy, that there are several channels at critical points in the body through which electricity can flow in and out in a constant stream. These are called the chakras.

The word chakra means 'wheel' in Sanskrit, although this is not like all the wheels we have seen. The chakra energy rotates clockwise as it moves the heat from our body to the field around us, and it rotates counterclockwise to draw power from our external world (and people). That integrate it) into our bodies. It is the recurrence condition of our chakras that decides in which heading our vitality will stream when they pull in or discharge energy into our body.

But are our chakras physical entities? Are they real wheels turning in the seven main centers of our body? No, They are not made of matter; They are energetic. But just like a fan's buzzing, it doesn't mean they aren't there just because you can't see them.

You may be thinking how it is possible for us to know if there are chakras if we cannot see them. It is a valid question for which science has not yet found a problematic answer. It was a breakthrough for me as a scientifically minded person when I started learning about chakra healing. I am a scientist, not a philosopher; it is the resistance that my ego threw at me when I began to explore what was a new frontier for me. But although the concept of chakras was new to me (and still manages to get around scientific evidence), it has been around for thousands of years and in different cultures.

It is something that I have '' demonstrated '' through my understanding and in my chakra mending work with my patients. The impact of our body's vitality, the existence power moving through this book, and the quality of the quantum field itself are things that have not yet outperformed our logical capacities. I genuinely believe that we will get there eventually, but until then, we can only trust our experience and the teachings of others.

We can additionally comprehend the fiery presence of our chakras (and their related feelings) by following their shading, which becomes essential in the chakra healing exercises that I will describe later in this article. Yes, each chakra has a corresponding color. Visible light emits electromagnetic waves, which move back and forth across the field through time and space. Depending on how fast the waves vibrate, our eyes will capture them in different colors. For example, red is a lower frequency wave that resembles a slow spin; The chakra energies, which vibrate at their different frequencies, also have different colors.

How does chakra work?

A chakra can be a wheel or a whirlpool, yet it works like a bundle of energy that enters the physical body. The chakras themselves are not physical; you can't see them on an x-shaft. They are parts of awareness and interface with the material and vigorous body through two essential vehicles, the endocrine framework, and the sensory system. Every one of the seven chakras is related to one of the nine endocrine organs, as well as a specific group of nerves called the plexus, making them essential elements in healing. Therefore, each chakra corresponds to certain parts of the body and particular functions in the body that are controlled by that plexus or endocrine gland, which is the key to understanding how the chakra healing methods work.

The chakras speak to specific pieces of your physical body, as well as particular parts of your awareness. Your cognizance, how you see your existence, speaks to all that you can understanding. The entirety of your faculties, recognitions, and potential conditions of information can be partitioned into seven classifications, and every one of these classes can be related to a specific chakra. At the point when you feel the pressure in your cognizance, you feel it in the chakra that has a place with the piece of your insight.

Open and close chakras.

Opening and closing our chakras work as an energetic defense system. A negative experience (and the accompanying low-frequency energy) can cause the associated chakra energy to shut down to block that energy. Similarly, we close the chakra (the channel through which heat would escape), if we hold onto a feeling of low calibration like guilt, we prolong the emotion because we refuse to deal with it or move it, creating a particular chakra. Healing techniques such as the Breath of Fire exercise described below are required. Any of the emotions at the bottom of the Quantum Lovemap (described in my book) are likely to cause a chakra energy restriction. I think we feel that tension as the tension that enters our mind and body when we are stressed.

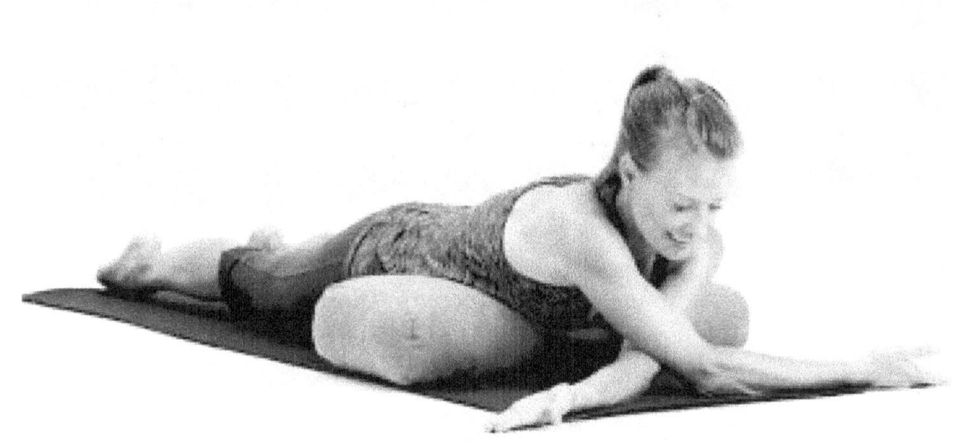

When we open and heal our chakras, the energy can flow freely again, and things return to normal. Sometimes it is about moving energy throughout our body, moving our frequency to the Quantum Love Map, or tackling and removing a painful spine that is causing us stress. For now, I just want you to understand the importance of chakra healing and that your chakras are open and allow energy to pass through you unobstructed. Any connection of chakras to a major endocrine gland and nervous system in your body means that a lack of energy can have serious physical consequences if you ignore it for too long. I often wonder if the heart pain I experienced when my mother died suppressed my immune system enough,
along with all the negative thinking, anxiety, and sugar (cancer cells have far more glucose receptors than healthy cells), cancer cells that were already in my body to grow.

Balance is critical in chakra healing.

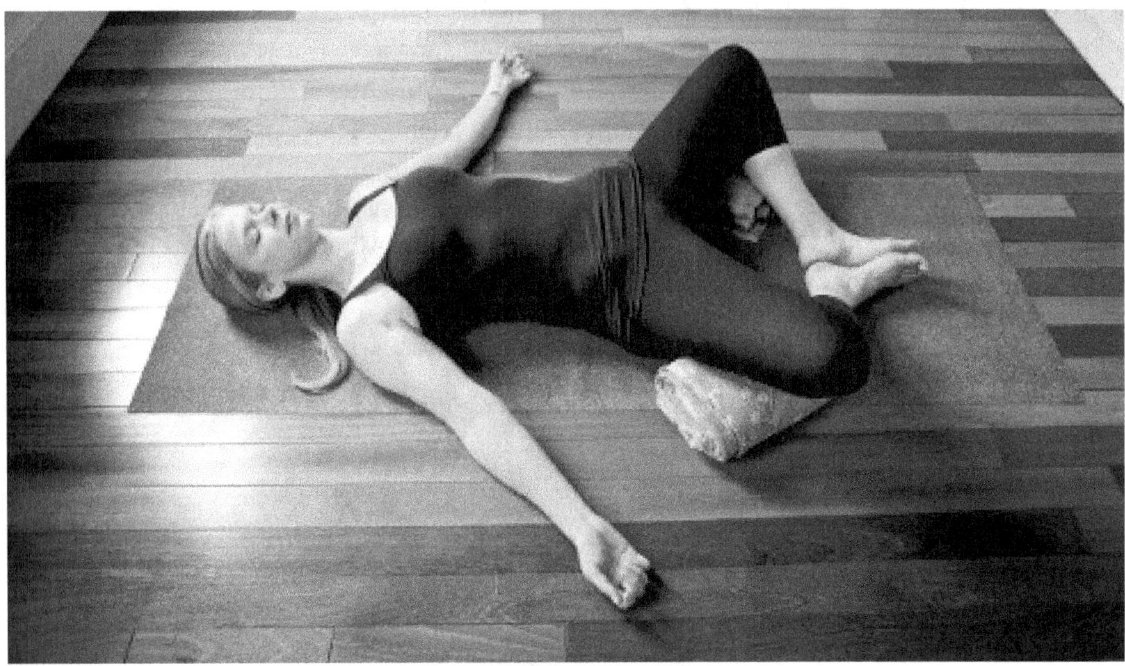

No chakra is better than the other or more important than any other in the process of body energy balance and chakra healing. You don't want extra heart chakra energy and less throat chakra energy; it just doesn't work that way. Ideally, all of your seven chakras are healed, balanced, open, and buzzing, allowing energy to flow in and out of your body. The fantastic thing is that your body is going to find a way to move the heat in and out (unless, of course, your ego tells you to clutch something).

Because your body wants to achieve an energy balance in your chakras, moving too far in any direction (inactive or hyperactive) in a chakra can cause adverse effects on your body and backfire on the energy body and the healing process, of the chakra. A slow chakra kicks another chakra into overdrive, which in turn draws additional energy from that part of the body. The descriptions below demonstrate how to act or feel when your chakras become unbalanced and need healing. The first gives a review of the physical frameworks related to each chakra and the conceivable physical side effects that may show that something isn't right.

How to keep the energy flowing
When energy is trapped in a particular chakra, make sure the weather flows through these tips:

1st chakra (root)

Element: The root chakra is associated with the ground, so walking barefoot in sand, grass, or dirt can be helpful. Any time in nature is useful for this chakra.
Diet: Eat healthy red foods like tomatoes, beets, berries, and apples.
Wear and Decorate: Wear red accents and wear red jewelry, clothing, or shoes.
Sound: lamb

2nd chakra (sacrum)

Element: The sacral chakra is associated with water, which means that it is beneficial to swim or spend time in streams such as lakes and oceans.
Diet: Eat orange foods like carrots, oranges, melons, or mangoes.
Use and decorate: Surround yourself with accessories or orange tones.
Sound: vam

3rd chakra (solar plexus)

Element: The solar plexus chakra is associated with the part of the fire, so enjoy sitting around a campfire or enjoying bright sunlight.
Diet: Eat yellow nourishments like bananas, ginger, turmeric, pineapple, and corn.
Wear and Decorate: Wearing yellow garments, gems, and adornments would be useful.
Sound: ram

4th chakra (heart)

Components: The heart chakra is related to air, so profound breathing will help scrub vitality at this level. Drive with the windows open, fly a kite, or take a vessel ride.
Diet: Eat green nourishments like broccoli, avocado, and verdant green vegetables like kale or spinach.
Utilize and design: complement your existence with all shades of green.
Sound: mmm

5th chakra (throat)

Component: The throat chakra is related to the ether (like the soul), so sitting in an open space under a reasonable sky is an incredible method to stream this vitality appropriately.
Diet: Eat blue nourishments like blueberries, gooseberries, mythical serpent natural products, and ocean growth.

Wear and enrich: utilize all shades of blue.
Sound: ham

6th chakra (third eye)

Component: The third eye chakra is related to light. To adjust and open this chakra, sit discreetly in the daylight or unwind in a window while the sun rises.Diet: Eat indigo foods such as purple kale, grapes, and blackberries.
Wearing and decorating: Wearing indigo clothing or jewelry and decorating with details of this color will be useful.
Sound: appearance

7th chakra (crown)

Element: The crown chakra is connected to all aspects, so it is a recommended practice to contact your integrity rather than a single item. Spend time meditating, singing, or praying.
Nutrition: At this level, diet is no longer for the physical body. This chakra is not fed with food, but with spiritual exercises—practice self-reflection and curiosity.
Wear and decorate: it will be useful to wear purple clothes or jewelry and decorate with details of this color.

6 Tips To Balance Your Chakras

1. colors

Let your intuition guide you when choosing the colors you want to use. All of our energy centers have a specific frequency that resonates with particular shades that have a similar rate. For example, if you don't

feel safe or grounded, your root chakra may be out of balance with the rest of your energy centers. You may be drawn to the use of red these days. Whether it's outerwear or underwear, this will help filter out the color you need to restore balance to the energy center.

2. to eat

Adjust your diet to include more foods with the same chakra color that you are trying to balance. Use the root chakra again as an example and try adding more red foods to your diet such as tomatoes, radishes, watermelons, bell peppers, pomegranates.

3. sound

Just as a color has a frequency, so makes music. Our energy centers resonate on specific musical notes.

Root = C, sacrum = D, solar plexus = E, heart = F, throat = G, third eye = A, crown = B. Listening to music on the notes above will stimulate that specific energy center (classical music is good enough for this).

4. reinforcement

We can also use our voice to create tones to stimulate and balance the energy centers. Place both hands on the unbalanced energy center, and then begin to sound your most profound possible ringtone, gradually increasing the pitch. You will intuitively know which shade is right for you as you will feel the center lighter and respond to that shade. Wear this shade all day/week until you feel more balanced.

5. Essential oils

Essential oils additionally reverberate at a particular recurrence and can be utilized to adjust the chakras. They can be applied directly or by inhalation. (If applied directly to the skin, make sure they are sufficiently diluted with a suitable carrier oil.)

6. Visualization

Visualization is perhaps the most powerful tool of all. While meditating, visualize that you are recovering energy from the center of the earth and cleaning each energy center, with the consistent color, sound, and frequency.

REDUCE ANXIETY

If you are anxious, you may be trapped and not know how to feel better. You can even do things that unconsciously awaken your fear. You could focus on the future and get carried away by a lot of hypothetical situations. How do you reduce your anxiety now?

What if I start to feel worse? What if they hate my presentation? What if he sees me sweating? What happens if I bomb the exam? What happens if I don't get the house? You could judge yourself and criticize your fear. You may think that your worst negative scenarios are indisputable facts. Fortunately, there are many tools and techniques that you can use to control anxiety effectively. Below, experts have shared healthy ways to deal with stress.

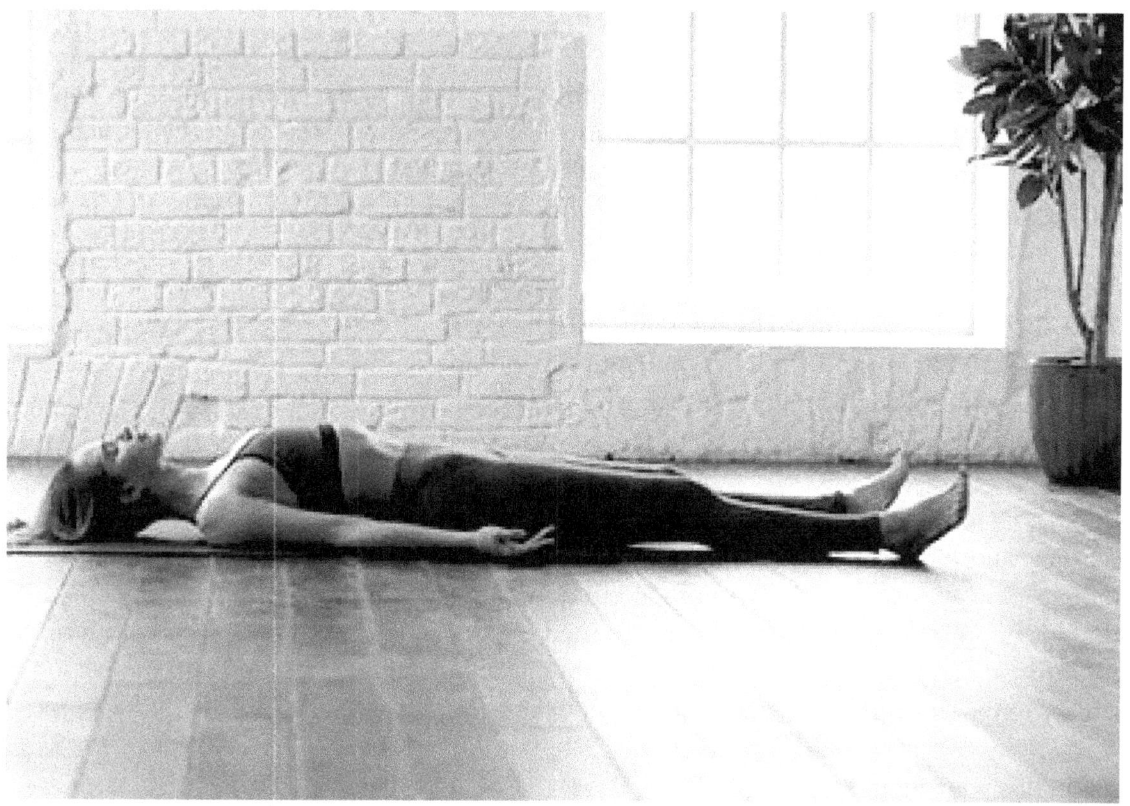

Now reduce anxiety symptoms
How do you now reduce or eliminate your anxiety and fear? Here are nine ways to do that
have been shown to work.

1. Take a deep breath.
"The principal thing you ought to do when you're on edge is to inhale," said Tom Corboy,
MFT, originator, and CEO of the Los Angeles OCD Center, and co-writer of the up and
coming book The Mindfulness Workbook for OCD. Profound diaphragmatic breathing is
a fantastic strategy for decreasing tension since it initiates the body's unwinding reaction.
It enables the body to move from the battle or-flight opinion of the thoughtful sensory system to the casual response of the parasympathetic sensory system, said Marla W. Deibler,
PsyD, clinical analyst, and chief of the Greater Philadelphia Center for Emotional Health. , LLC.

She proposed this activity: "Attempt to breathe in gradually until you check 4, first filling
your stomach area and afterward your chest, delicately holding your breath until you tally
four and breathing out gradually until you tally four and rehash a few times."

2. Accept that you are afraid

Acceptance is critical because trying to combat or eliminate anxiety often makes it worse.
It just continues the idea that your fear is unbearable, he said. But accepting your fear
does not mean that you like or resign yourself to a miserable existence.
"It merely means that you would benefit if you accepted reality as it is, and at that moment, reality includes fear.

3. Realize that your brain is cheating on you.
Psychiatrist Kelli Hyland, M.D., has seen first-hand how someone's brain can make them
believe they are dying of a heart attack while having a panic attack. He recalled an experience he had gained as a medical student.

Some people who had heart attacks and looked so sick on medical floors for medical
reasons, and they looked the same. A wise, kind and experienced psychiatrist came to [the
patient] and gently and calmly reminded him that he will not die, that it will happen, and
that his brain is deceiving him. He also calmed me down, and we both stayed with him
until [the panic attack] ended. "'It helps eliminate shame, guilt, pressure, and the responsibility to repair or judge yourself when you need care more than ever."

4. Discuss your thoughts.

"When people are anxious, their brains begin to have all kinds of strange ideas, many of which are very unrealistic and unlikely to occur," said Corboy. And these thoughts only reinforce a person's state of anxiety. Let's say you are about to make a wedding toast. Thoughts like, "Oh my gosh, I can't do this. It will kill me," you might go through your head.

Remember, though, this is not a disaster, and no one died while toasting, Corboy said. "Yes, you may be scared, and you may even drop your toast. But the worst that will happen is that some people, many of whom will never see you again, laugh and forget about it tomorrow. '
Deibler additionally proposed asking yourself these inquiries while testing your musings:

* 	Is this worry reasonable?
* 	Will this happen?
* 	If the worst outcome were to occur, what would be wrong?
* 	Could you handle that?
* 	What am I supposed to do?
* 	If something terrible happens, what can it mean for me?
* 	Is this true, or does it seem wt?

5. Use a relaxing visualization.
Hyland suggested practicing the following meditation regularly, making it easier to access if you are anxious at the time. Imagine yourself standing on the riverbank or outside in a favorite park, field, or beach. Watch the leaves go by the river or the clouds.

This is very different from what people usually do. Most of the time, we assign emotions, thoughts, and physical sensations to certain qualities and judgments, such as right or wrong, right or wrong, Hyland said. And this often reinforces fear. Remember that "everything is just information."

6. Be an observer without judgment.
"Practice perception (considerations, sentiments, feelings, sensations, judgment) with empathy or without judgment." "I have had patients returned after months or years, and they said they, despite everything, have that map on their mirror or the dashboard of their vehicle, and it causes them."
7. Use positive internal dialogue.
Anxiety can cause a lot of negative talks. Say to yourself "positive coping statements," Deibler said. For example, you might say, "This fear feels bad, but I can use strategies to deal with it."

8. Now focus on.
"When people are anxious, they are generally obsessed with something that could happen in the future," Corboy said. Instead, pause, breathe, and watch what's going on right now, he said. Even if something serious happens, focusing on the present moment will improve your ability to handle the situation, he added.

9. Focus on meaningful activities.
If you're feeling anxious, it's also helpful to direct your attention to "meaningful and helpful activity," Corboy said. He suggested wondering what he would do if he weren't afraid. If you saw a movie, still watch. If you are going to do laundry, do it.

"The worst thing you can do when you're anxious is to be passively obsessed with how you feel." Doing what needs to be done teaches you valuable lessons, he said: getting out of your head feels better; you can live your life even if you are anxious, and you do things 'The bottom line is: be busy with life issues. Don't focus on anxiety; nothing good will come of it. "

LOW-STRESS LEVELS

Here we might want to begin by giving you a prologue to what stress is, what are the indications of stress, what basic strides to take on the off chance that you are feeling focused, and practical tips to avoid it, to show why we are passionate about moving to a less stressed nation.

What is stress?

Stress is the inclination of being feeling the squeeze. This weight can emerge out of various parts of your everyday life.. Like an increased workload, a transition period, an argument with your family, or new and existing financial concerns. You may notice that it has a cumulative effect, with each stressor building on top each other. During these circumstances, you may feel compromised or upset, and your body may cause a pressure reaction. This can cause an assortment of physical manifestations, change how you act, and cause you to encounter increasingly exceptional feelings.

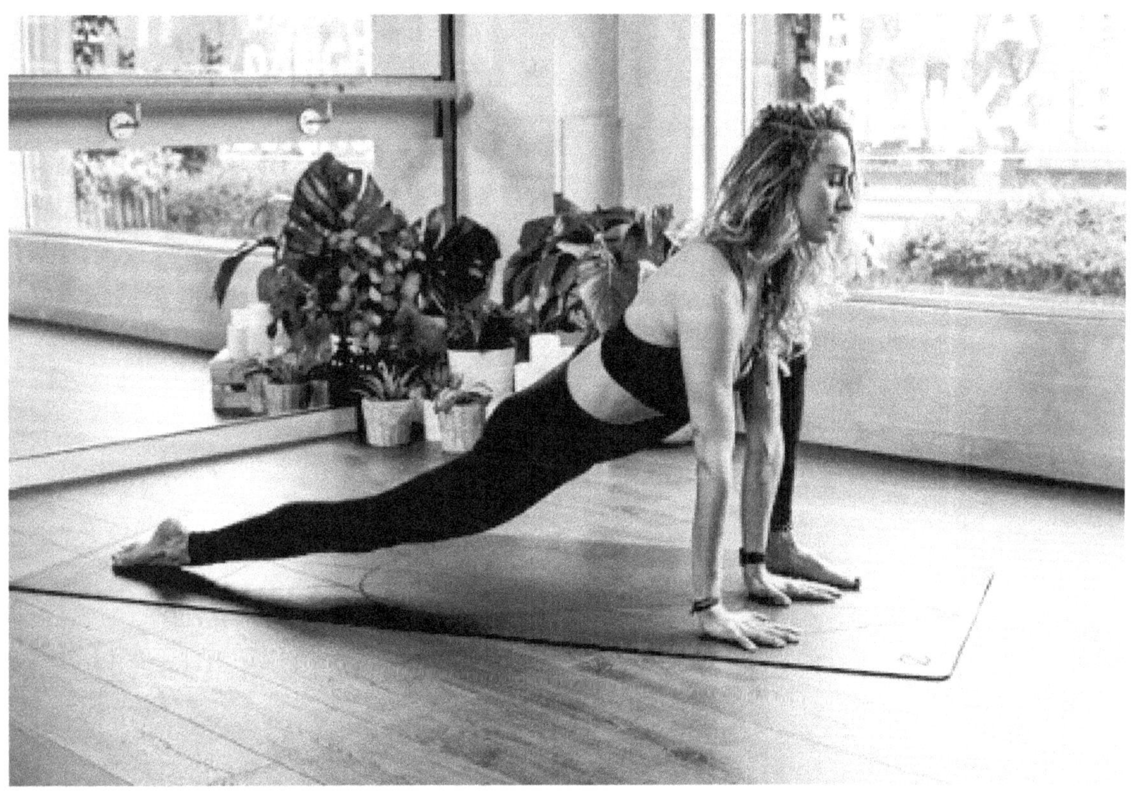

Stress affects us in various ways, both physically and emotionally, and at different intensities.

How can I recognize the signs of stress?
Everyone experiences stress. However, if it affects your life, health, and well-being, it is essential to address it as soon as possible, and although stress affects everyone differently, there are common signs and symptoms to consider: 15

- feelings of constant worry or fear
- feelings of being overwhelmed
- difficult to focus
- mood swings or changes in your mood
- irritability or short temper
- difficulty relaxing
- depression
- low self-esteem
- eat more or less than normal
- changes in your sleep habits
- use alcohol, tobacco, or illegal drugs to relax
- aches and pains, especially muscle tension
- diarrhea and constipation
- nausea or dizziness
- Loss of sexual desire.

If you experience these symptoms for a long time and think they affect your daily life or feel unwell, contact your doctor. You can request information about the supportive services and treatments available to you.

Three steps to take when you're stressed

1. Realize when you're causing a problem
- Sick and the pressure you face
- Watch out for physical warnings like tight muscles, fatigue, headaches, or migraines

2. Identify the causes.
- Try to identify the underlying causes
- Classify the possible reasons for your stress into three categories 1) those that have a practical solution 2) those that improve over time and 3) those that you cannot avoid
- Try to release and let go of the concerns of those in the second and third groups.

3. Review your lifestyle
•	Can you assume too much?
•	Are there things you do that can be transferred to someone else?
•	Can you do things in a more relaxed way?
•	To answer the answers to these questions, you may need to prioritize the things you are trying to accomplish and reorganize your life.
•	This will help ease the pressure that can come from trying to do everything at once.

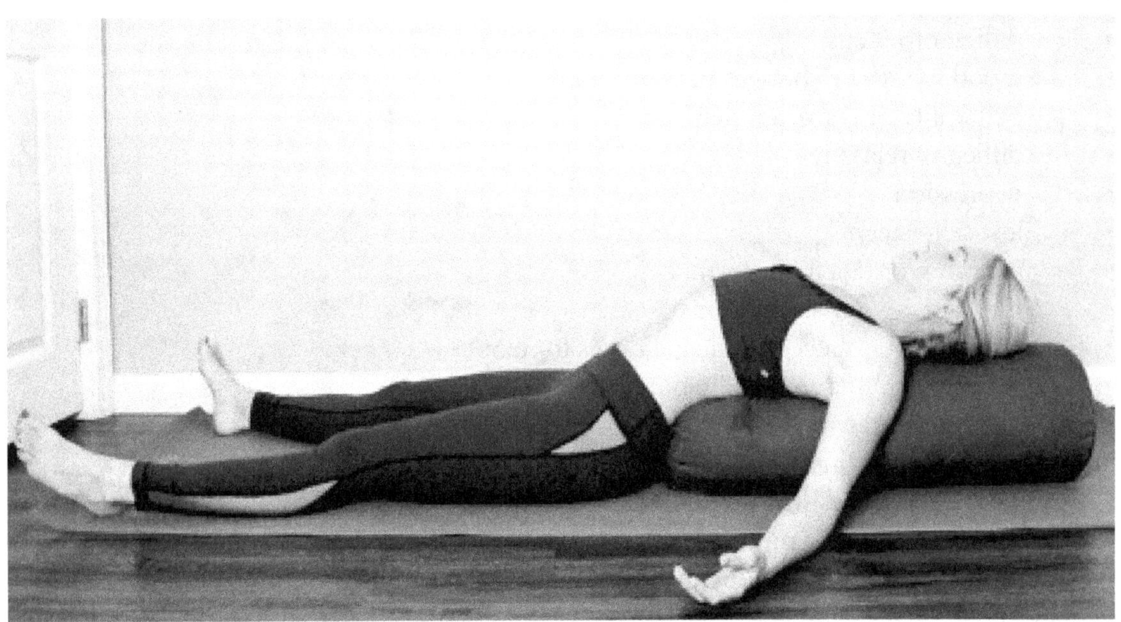

Seven steps to protect yourself from stress

1. Eat healthily
Eating healthy can reduce the risks of diet-related illnesses39
There is increasing evidence showing how food affects our mood40 and how a healthy diet can improve it.
You can protect your sense of well-being by ensuring that your diet contains satisfactory measures of mind supplements, for example, fundamental nutrients and minerals, just as water

2. Be careful with smoking and drinking alcohol.
Do not try or reduce the amount you smoke and drink alcohol.

Although they initially seem to relieve tension, this is misleading as they often exacerbate problems42

3. Exercise
Try to integrate training into your lifestyle, as it can be beneficial in reducing stress.
Even going out and getting some fresh air and doing some light exercise, like walking to the store, can help43

4. Take some time relax
Find the balance between responsibility for others and responsibility for yourself; this can reduce stress levels.
Tell yourself that prioritizing self-care is okay. · You need a wait time, but say, "I can't take a break," then read more about how taking a break is essential to good mental health professional. Health

5. Keep in mind
Care is a brain-body way to deal with life that causes us to manage encounters unexpectedly. It includes focusing on our considerations and emotions in a manner that improves our capacity to deal with unpleasant circumstances and settle on savvy choices. Try to practice mindfulness regularly
Mindfulness meditation can be practiced anywhere, anytime
Research has shown that it can reduce the effects of stress, anxiety, and related problems, such as insomnia, lack of concentration, and bad mood in some people.
Our Be Mindful website offers a specially developed online mindfulness course as well as details of local classes in your area.

6. Sleep easy
Do you think you are sleeping?
Can your physical or mental health affect your ability to sleep?
Can you adjust your environment to improve your sleep?
Can you get up instead of staying in bed if you are worried at night?
Can you make small lifestyle changes to get a good night's sleep?

7. Don't be too hard on yourself
Try to keep things in perspective.
Remember that a bad day is a universal human experience.

If your internal critic or an external critic discovers mistakes, try to find the truth and an exception to what is said
If you stumble or think you have failed, don't hit yourself
Pretend to be your own best friend: be kind and caring

What can long-term stress lead to?
Stress is a natural response to many life situations, such as work, family, relationships, and money problems.
We mentioned earlier that a moderate amount of stress could help us perform better in stressful situations, 34, but excessive or prolonged stress can lead to physical problems. This may include lower levels of immunity, digestive and intestinal problems, e.g , peevish entrail disorder (IBS) 36 or emotional well-being issues, for example, misery. This implies it is fundamental to control pressure and keep it at a stable level to stay away from long haul harm to the body and brain.

Some common symptoms of stress are difficulty sleeping, sweating, or a change in appetite 6,7.Symptoms like this are caused by an increase in stress hormones in your body, which, when released, allows you to deal with pressure or threats. Hormones called adrenaline and norepinephrine increase blood pressure, increase heart rate, and increase the rate at which you sweat.

This prepares your body for an emergency. These hormones can also decrease blood flow to your skin and reduce stomach action. Cortisol, another pressure hormone, discharges fat, and sugar into your framework to build your vitality. Thus, you may encounter migraines, muscle strain, torment, queasiness, acid reflux, and unsteadiness. You can also breathe faster, have palpitations, or experience various aches and pains. In the long run, you may be at risk for heart attacks and strokes.

All of these changes are how your body makes it easier for you to fight or flight, and once the pressure or threat is over, your stress hormone levels will generally return to normal. However, if you are consistently low stress, these hormones remain in the body and cause the symptoms of anxiety In case you're stuck in a bustling office. or on a crowded train, you can't fight or escape, so you can't use the chemicals your own body produces to protect you. Over time, the accumulation of these chemicals and the changes they cause can be harmful to your health.

What are the behavioral and emotional effects of stress?
When you're stressed, you can experience many different feelings, such as anxiety, irritability, or low self-esteem, which can cause you to withdraw, become indecisive, and cry.

You may encounter times of consistent stress, hustling musings,
 or repeated thoughts about the same things in your head. You may experience changes in
your behavior. You may lose control more easily, act irrationally, or become more verbal
or physically aggressive.14 These feelings can feed each other and cause physical symptoms that can exacerbate you feel even. For instance, excessive tension can cause you to
feel so awful. that you worry that you are in serious physical condition.

What causes stress?
All kinds of situations can cause stress. The most common are work, money, and relationships with partners, children, or other family members. Stress can be caused by significant
disorders and life events such as divorce, unemployment, movement, and pain, or a series
of minor irritations, such as feeling undervalued at work or arguing with a family mem-
ber.16 Sometimes there are no apparent causes.

Relationships and stress
Relationships are very supportive in times of stress. But from time to time, people close to
you, be it a partner, parent, child, friend, or colleague, can increase your stress levels.

Money and stress
Money and debt put enormous pressure on us, so it is not surprising that they have a
definite effect on our stress levels. The consequences of the economic crisis, in one way or
another, have affected everyone. Recent StepChange Debt Charity statistics found a 56%
increase in demand for debt advice and support from 2012-2014.23 Citizens Advice saw
a similar increase in the number of people suffering from finances and facing 6,407 debt
problems every year. business days 24

A 2013 survey found that 42% of those seeking debt help had prescription drugs from
their primary care physician to help them deal with them, while 76% of people in a couple said debt affected their relation.

Smoking, drinking and using drugs and stress
You can smoke, drink alcohol, or use recreational drugs to reduce stress. However,
this often worsens the problems. Research shows that smoking can increase feelings of
anxiety.29 Nicotine provides an immediate and temporary sense of relaxation, which can
subsequently lead to withdrawal symptoms and cravings.
Similarly, you can use alcohol as a means of dealing with and coping with painful feelings and to temporarily reduce feelings of anxiety. However, alcohol can worsen existing
psychological problems. It can cause you to feel progressively on edge and discouraged in
the long run. It is essential to know the suggested limits and drink capably.

Physician recommended meds, for example, sedatives and resting tablets, which may have to endorsed for phenomenal reasons, can likewise cause mental and physical medical issues whenever utilized for a long time.32 Street drugs, for example, cannabis or Ecstasy, are commonly taken for recreational purposes. For specific individuals, issues start when their bodies become acclimated to rehashed utilization of the medication. This leads to higher doses to maintain the same effect.

How can you help yourself?
Stress is a natural response to many life situations, such as work, family, relationships, and money problems.
We mentioned earlier that a moderate amount of stress could help us perform better in stressful situations, 34, but excessive or prolonged stress can lead to physical problems. This may include lower levels of immunity, digestive and intestinal problems, e.g., irritable bowel syndrome (IBS) 36 or mental health problems like depression.37 Therefore;
We must control our stress and keep it at a healthy level to avoid long-term damage to our body and mind.

Don't forget to seek help and support when you need it.
Recollect that it is alright to request expert guidance. If you have an inclination that you are making some hard memories getting by all alone, you can connect. It is essential to realize that you can find support as quickly as time permits and that you merit improvement.

The principal individual you approach is your primary care physician. The person in question ought to have the option to prompt you on treatment and allude you to another neighborhood proficient. Subjective conduct treatment (this is a kind of therapy that encourages you to comprehend that your contemplations and activities can influence how you feel) and care based methodologies help decrease pressure. A few voluntary associations can assist you with tending to the reasons for stress and prompt you on the most proficient method to improve.

INCREASE FLEXIBILITY

What every yoga should know about flexibility
While yoga isn't generally about being increasingly adaptable, understanding what adaptability is, and why it's significant can assist you with taking your yoga practice to the following level. If you are already practicing yoga, you don't need exercise scientists and physiologists to convince yourself of the benefits of stretching. Instead, you probably want to be told if there is anything in your flexibility research that can help you dig deeper into your asanas. For example, if science folds forward and the tension in the back of your legs keeps you short, can science tell you what's going on? And that knowledge can help you dig deeper?

The response to the two inquiries is "Yes." Knowledge of physiology can assist you with envisioning the internal activities of your body and spotlight on the particular systems that help you stretch. You can upgrade your endeavors by knowing whether the strain in your legs is the consequence of skeletal misalignment, inflexible connective tissues, or nerve reflexes intended to dodge injury. And if you know if any unpleasant feelings you are feeling are a warning that you are about to hurt, or Whether you find yourself entering exciting new territory, you can make a smart choice between pushing backward or backward, and preventing injury.

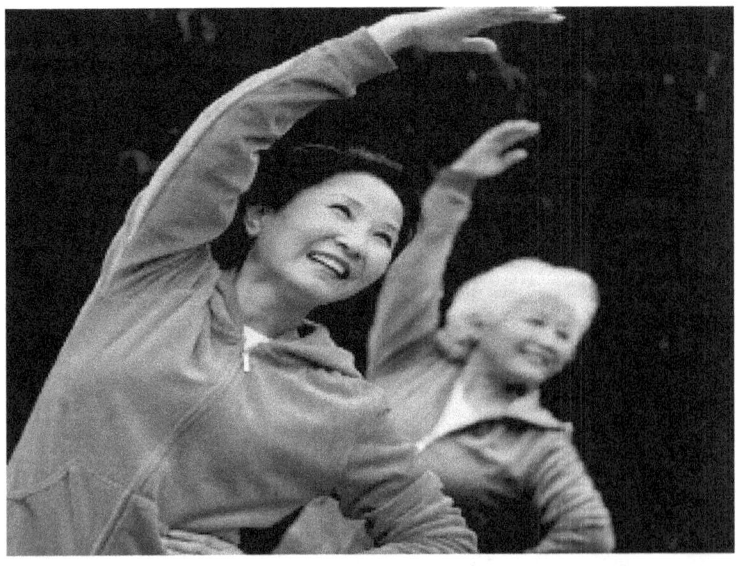

Understanding flexibility
In the study of flexibility, we deal with three types of connective tissue: tendons, ligaments, and muscle fascia. Yoga, of course, does much more than keep us agile. It releases the tension of our body and mind, allowing us to deepen our meditation. In yoga, "flexibility" is an attitude that inverts and transforms both the mind and the body.

Flexibility and musculature
Muscles are organs: natural units made up of different specific tissues that are coordinated to play out an individual capacity. (Physiologists segment muscles into three sorts: the smooth muscles of the viscera; the specific cardiovascular muscles of the heart; and the striated muscles of the skeleton, anyway at present, the inside just around the skeletal muscles, which are known pulleys that switch. bones of our body)

The particular capacity of muscles is the development created by muscle filaments, specific cell packages that change shape when contracting or unwinding. Muscle bunches cooperate, substitute, and stretch in particular, facilitated courses of action to deliver a full scope of developments that our bodies can do.

In skeletal developments, the muscles that work (the muscles that agreement to move the bones) are designated "agonists." Different muscle gatherings, the muscles that should be discharged and protracted to permit development, are classified "rivals." Almost all skeletal changes include the planned activity of agonist and foe muscle gatherings: they are the yang and yin of our development life systems.

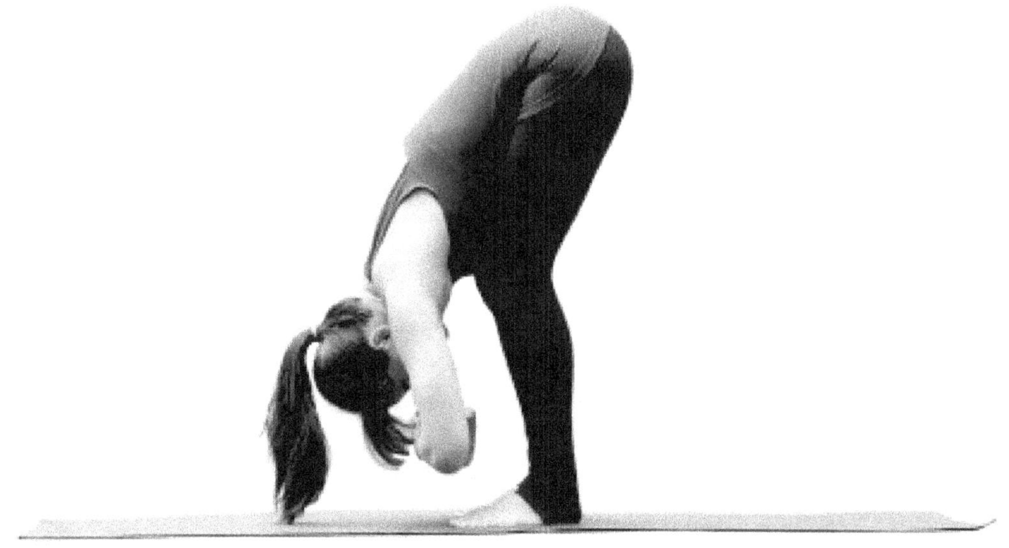

What limits flexibility?
If your muscle fibers don't limit your stretching ability, what will? There are two primary
science schools on what limits flexibility the most and what needs to be done to improve it.
The principal school centers not around extending muscle filaments,
but on increasing the elasticity of connective tissues, encapsulating and connecting the
cells that link muscle fibers to other organs; the second deals with the "stretch reflex" and
other functions of the autonomic (involuntary) nervous system. Yoga works on both. This
is why it is such an effective method of increasing flexibility.

Connective tissues comprise a variety of cell groups that specialize in uniting and it forms
a complex network that connects all our body parts and divides them into separate packages of anatomical structure: bones, muscles, organs, etc. Almost all yoga asanas practice
and improve their cellular quality in a varied way. And vital tissue, which transmits movement and supplies our muscles with ointments and mending specialists. However, in the
investigation of adaptability, we are keen on just three kinds of connective tissue: ligaments, tendons, and muscle belt. We should investigate every one of them.
Tendons transmit force by connecting bones to muscles. They are relatively rigid. If not,
excellent motor coordination, like playing the piano or eye surgery, would be impossible.
Although tendons have tremendous tensile strength, they have poor stretch tolerance.
After a 4 percent stretch, the muscles can rupture or grow beyond their recoil ability,
giving us lax and less sensitive muscle-bone connections.

Ligaments can safely stretch a little more than tendons, but not much. Ligaments tie issue
that remains to be worked out in joint cases. They assume a helpful job in restricting
adaptability, and it is by and large prescribed not to extend them.Stretching the ligaments
can destabilize the joints, compromise their efficiency, and increase the risk of injury. Therefore, you should bend your knees slightly, rather than exaggerate, in Paschimottanasana
(Seated Forward Bend), which reduces strain on the bands of the rear knees (and also the
ligaments of the lower back).

Muscular fascia is the third connective tissue that affects the flexibility and, by far, the
most important. Fascia represents up to 30 percent of a muscle's total mass, and according to studies cited in Science of Flexibility, it represents approximately 41 percent of a
muscle's overall resistance to movement. Fascia is the material that separates individual
muscle fibers and groups them into work units, providing structure and transmission
power.

How long does it stretch to increase flexibility
In these types of exercises, you maintain your posture long enough to affect the plastic quality of your connective tissue. Long stretching exercises like this can lead to permanent and healthy changes in the quality of the fascia that joins the muscles. Julie Gudmestad, a certified physical therapist and instructor at Iyengar, uses long-term asanas on patients at her clinic in Portland, Oregon. "If they hold the postures for shorter periods, people will have a good feeling of release," explains Gudmestad, "but they won't necessarily get the structural changes that lead to a permanent increase in flexibility."

According to Gudmestad, stretching exercises should be performed for 90 to 120 seconds to change the "soil substance" of the connective tissue. The ground powder is a gel-like, non-fibrous binder incorporating fibrous connective tissues such as collagen and elastin. Soil dust stabilizes and lubricates the connective tissue. What's more, it's by, and abundant accepted that impediments on this substance could restrain adaptability, particularly as we age.

Mutual flexibility and inhibition.
In addition to stretching the connective tissue, much of the work we do in yoga focuses on engaging the neurological mechanisms that allow our muscles to loosen and expand. One of those mechanisms is "mutual inhibition." Every time a set of muscles (the agonists) contract, this built-in feature of the autonomic nervous system releases the opposing muscles (the antagonists). Yogis have been using this mechanism for thousands of years to facilitate stretching exercises.

To experience mutual inhibition firsthand, sit down at a table, and gently press the edge of your karate chop style hand onto the table. If you touch the upper part of the upper arm, the triceps muscle, you will notice that it is firmly attached. When you reach the opposite muscles, the biceps (the large muscles at the front of the upper arm) should feel relaxed.

The same mechanism plays in Paschimottanasana. Your hamstrings are released when you activate your different muscle group, the quadriceps.

David Sheer, a manual orthopedic therapist in Nashville, Tennessee, uses the principle of mutual inhibition to help patients improve their range of motion safely. If you went to Sheer to enhance the flexibility of your hamstrings, he would train the quads and develop strength in the front of the thigh to relax the hamstrings. When the hamstrings have reached their maximum range for the day, Sheer will strengthen them with isometric or isotonic exercises that support the weight.

"I remind my students to put their quads together," says Larson, "and he lifts the entire length from the front of the leg so that the back of the leg comes off." Larson also includes backbends in his classes to strengthen the hamstrings and backs of his students. You need to develop strength in the muscles you are stretching. Like many teachers, Larson uses ancient yoga techniques that apply physiological principles that have only recently been understood by modern science.

According to Sheer, she is doing the right thing. He claims that the best kind of flexibility combines an improved range of motion with enhanced strength. "It's useful flexibility," says Sheer. "If you just increase your passive flexibility without developing the strength to control it, you will become more vulnerable to serious joint injury."
You can't go deeper into the posture as you would like, and the more you try, the tighter your hamstrings will feel. Then your instructor will remind you to continue breathing and relax any muscles that are not actively maintaining the pose.

You give up to match your best personal brand. You relax without judging the pose and slowly begin to release your hamstrings.

To get an idea of the stretch reflex, imagine walking through a winter landscape. Suddenly you stand on a piece of ice, and your feet begin to crumble. Immediately his muscles kick in, tense to bring his legs together, and regain control. What just happened to your nerves and muscles?

Each muscle fiber has a network of sensors called muscle coils. They run perpendicular to the muscle fibers and feel how far and quickly the fibers stretch as the muscle fibers lengthen, the tension in these muscle coils increases.

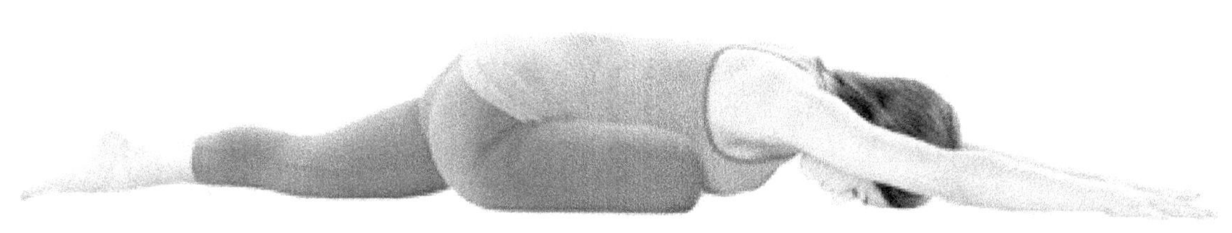

When this stress appears too fast or goes too far, the muscle coils trigger an urgent neuro-logical "SOS" that triggers a reflex loop that causes an immediate protective contraction.

That is what happens when the doctor hits a small rubber mallet on the tendon just below the kneecap and abruptly stretches the quads. This fast stretch invigorates the muscle ax-les in the quadriceps and signs the spinal rope. Moments later, the neurological loop ends with a brief contraction of the quadriceps, causing the well-known "instinctive response."

In this way, the stretch reflex protects your muscles. And that's why most experts warn against bouncing while stretching. Bouncing on and off a shelf causes rapid stimulation of the muscle coils that generate reflex hardening and can increase the risk of injury.

Slow, static stretching also causes the stretch reflex, but not so abruptly. When you fold forward in Paschimottanasana, the muscle spindles in your hamstrings begin to demand resistance, creating tension in the muscles you are trying to stretch. Therefore, improving flexibility through static stretching takes a long time. The improvement comes from the slow conditioning of the muscle coils, training them to tolerate more tension before the neuro brakes are applied.

PNF and flexibility

Recent advances in western flexibility training include neurological techniques that retrain the stretch reflex and promote rapid and dramatic gains in flexibility. One of these techniques is called proprioceptive neuromuscular facilitation: take a deep breath. (Fortunately, it's usually just called PNF.)
To apply PNF principles to Paschimottanasana, try the following: While leaning forward, just before your maximum stretch, hold the hamstrings in an isometric contraction as if you are trying to pull your heels across the floor.

The PNF technique controls the stretch reflex by permitting you to get a muscle nearly to its most extreme length.. When you compromise your hamstrings, you relieve the pressure on your muscle pills and send signals that the flesh is sure to release even more. In an apparent paradox, the contraction of the muscle causes it to lengthen. If you turn on and then release your muscle fibers in this way, you're likely to find more comfort in a stretch that was almost its maximum a few seconds earlier. You are now ready to open up a bit more, using a momentary pause in neural activity, deepening the stretch. Your nervous system adjusts, giving you more freedom of movement.

"PNF is as close as we've come to logical extending," says physiotherapist Michael Leslie. Leslie utilizes blends of changed PNF methods to help individuals from the San Francisco Ballet improve their adaptability. "As far as I can tell, it can take a long time of static preparing to procure the potential gains in a PNF meeting.
Until now, yoga has not systematically focused on techniques similar to PNF. But vinyasa exercises that emphasize careful ordering of the asanas and repetition of the asanas, moving in and out of the same posture multiple times, tend to promote neurological conditioning.

How breathing helps increase flexibility
Kraftsow also emphasizes the importance of breathing in any type of neurological work, noting that breath is a connection between our cognizance and our autonomic sensory system. "It is this quality of respiration," says Kraftsow, "that makes it a primary tool in any science of self-development."

Pranayama, or breath control, is the fourth piece of a yogi's way to samadhi. One of the fundamental yoga rehearses enables the yogi to control the development of prana (imperative vitality) all through the body. Through complex yoga physiology or logical physiology in the West, the association between unwinding, extending, and breathing is entrenched. Physiologists depict this mechanical and neurological relationship of development and breath, for instance, of synkinesis, the automatic construction of one piece of the body that happens with the difference in another part.

As you hold Paschimottanasana and breathe deeply and continuously, you may notice an ebb and flow towards your stretch that reflects the tide of your breathing. As you breathe, your muscles tense slightly, reducing stretching. As you exhale, slowly and ultimately, your abdomen moves back to your spine, the muscles in your lower back seem to lengthen, and you can lower your chest to your thighs.

Exhalation deflates the lungs and lifts the diaphragm toward the chest, creating space in the abdominal cavity and facilitating forward flexion of the lumbar spine (Inward breath does the inverse, filling the stomach cavity like an inflatable, making it hard to twist the spine forward.) But you may not realize that exhaling also relaxes your back muscles and tilts your pelvis forward.

In Paschimottanasana, the muscles of the lower back are in latent strain. As per exa-mine referred to in Science of Flexibility, each inhalation is accompanied by an active contraction of the lower back, a decrease in direct contrast to the desired forward curve. Then exhalation releases the muscles of the lower back, facilitating stretching. By placing your palms on your back, just above your hips, and breathing deeply, you can feel the spinal erector on either side of the spine as you inhale and release as you exhale. If you pay close consideration, you will likewise see that with every inward breath, the muscles around the tailbone, at the tip of your spine, pull the pelvis slightly back. Each exhalation relaxes these muscles and frees the pelvis, allowing it to rotate around the hip joints.

As your lungs are empty and the diaphragm rises in your chest, your back muscles are released, and you can stretch to the limit. Once there, you can experience a seemingly eternal, pleasant moment of inner peace, where calming the nervous system has traditio-nally been considered one of the benefits of forwarding leaning.

At this point, you can feel especially in touch with the spiritual element of yoga. But we-stern science also provides a material explanation for this experience. As per Alter Flexi-bility Science, the stomach pushes against the heart during exhalation, bringing down the pulse. Circulatory strain diminishes, as stresses on the rib restrict, stomach dividers, and intercostal muscles. Unwinding creates, and your resistance to extending increments, as does your feeling of prosperity.

Shortcuts to flexibility

Not all moments in yoga are peaceful. At the end of hatha yoga performance, practitioners may experience breakthroughs that may involve some degree of pain, anxiety, and risk. (Hatha means "powerful" after all.) You may have seen the photo in B.K.S.'s Light on Yoga. Iyengar was standing in Mayurasana (peacock pose) on the back of a student in Paschimottanasana, forcing her to bend deeper. Or you may have seen a teacher standing on the thighs of a student in Baddha Konasana (Bound Angle Pose). Such methods may seem dangerous or even cruel to a stranger. Still, in the hands of an experienced instructor, they can be remarkably effective and bear a striking resemblance to advanced techniques in Western flexibility training that focus on restoring neurological mechanisms.

While researching this article, a friend told me about a time when he accidentally used one of these mechanisms and made a surprising breakthrough after years of trying to master Hanumanasana (a pose better known in the West as 'the splits'). One day when my friend tried the pose: his left leg forward and his right leg back, his hands lightly resting on the ground, he stretched his legs out more than usual, carrying almost the entire weight of his torso by his hips He stretched his legs out more than usual, allowing most of the importance of his body to rest on his hips. Suddenly she felt intense heat in her pelvic area and a sudden, sudden shock that brought her bones to the ground. My friend had caused a physiological reaction rarely found during stretching, a neurological 'circuit breaker' that counteracts and pushes the stretch reflex aside. While the stretch reflex tightens muscle tissue, this other reflex, technically known as the 'reverse myotatic reflex (stretch),' completely releases muscle tension to protect the tendons.

How it works At the ends of each muscle, where the fascia and tendons are intertwined, there are sensory bodies that follow the load. These are the Golgi Tendon Organs (GTO). They respond when a muscle contraction or stretch puts too much stress on a tendon. The state-sponsored mass sports team from the former Soviet Union developed a neurological flexibility training method mainly based on the manipulation of this GTO reflex. "You already have the muscle length you need," argues Russian flexibility expert Pavel Tsatsouline, "enough for full divisions and more difficult asanas. But to control flexibility, you need to master an autonomous function." Tsatsouline makes the point by raising her leg on a backrest. "If you can do this," he says, "you already have enough stretch to do the splits." According to Tsatsouline, muscle or connective tissue does not stop you. "Great flexibility can be achieved," says Tsatsouline, "by moving a few switches in the spinal cord."

But using the GTO mechanism to increase flexibility carries certain risks because the muscles must be fully expanded and under extreme stress to trigger a GTO reflex.

Implementing improved flexibility training methods, such as the Russian system or advanced yoga techniques, requires an experienced teacher who can ensure that your skeleton is aligned correctly and that your body is strong enough to handle stress. If you don't know what you are doing, you can easily injure yourself. However, when used correctly, these methods can be instrumental. Tsatsouline claims that she can teach even stiff middle-aged men without prior flexibility training, how to do the splits in about six months.

Yoga flexibility and philosophy.
Now you may be wondering, "What do these western stretching techniques have to do with yoga?"

On the one hand, stretching is, of course, an essential part of building yoga deha, the yoga body with which the practitioner channels more and more prana. That is one reason why the colossal hatha yoga schools base their training on traditional asanas, a progression of stances that represent and advance the entire scope of human development. In any case, any great educator will likewise reveal to you that yoga isn't just about extending. "Yoga is an order that shows us better approaches to encounter the world," Judith Lasater, Ph.D., and a physical specialist, he clarifies, "with the goal that we can surrender our connection to our anguish." According to Lasater, there are just two asanas: cognizant or oblivious. What recognizes a specific situation as an asana is our center, not merely the outside state of the body.

It is certainly possible to get so caught up in the pursuit of physical perfection that we lose sight of the "purpose" of asana practice: the state of samadhi. At the same time, however, exploring the limits of body flexibility can be a perfect way to develop concentration at one point necessary for the "inner limbs" of classical yoga.
Some yogis are already enthusiastically embracing this synthesis. At the Meridian Stretching Center in Boston, Massachusetts, Bob Cooley develops and tests a computer program that can diagnose flexibility deficits and prescribe asanas. New customers at Cooley's Stretch Center are asked to adopt 16 different yoga poses, as Cooley captures specific anatomical landmarks on their bodies with a digitizer wand, similar to the one used in computer-aided drawing. These body point measurements are calculated to make comparisons between the client and the average and maximum human flexibility models. The computer program generates a report that compares and guides the client's progress, describes areas for improvement and recommends specific asanas.

Cooley utilizes a combination of what he sees as the best purposes of eastern and western information, joining old-style yoga asana with systems like PNF.

If you are a yoga perfectionist, you dislike the possibility of a yoga variety, which consolidates new logical experiences with traditional yoga rehearses. In any case, "better than ever" has consistently been one of America's national mantras, and the best of Eastern trial knowledge and Western diagnostic science can be a fundamental commitment our nation makes to the advancement of yoga.

Yoga does typically substantially more than keep us agile. It discharges the strain of our body and brain, permitting us to develop our contemplation. In yoga, "adaptability" is a demeanor that upsets and changes both the mind and the body. Be that as it may, in western physiological terms, "adaptability" is only the capacity to move muscles and joints all through their range. It is the expertise brought into the world with, yet the more significant part of us lose. "Our lives are restricted and stationary," clarifies Dr. Thomas Green, a chiropractor in Lincoln, Nebraska, "with the goal that our bodies become sluggish, muscle decay and our joints are in a restricted range."

When we were hunter-gatherers, we received the daily exercise we needed to keep our bodies flexible and healthy. But modern and sedentary life is not the only culprit that contracts muscles and joints. Even when active, your body will dry out and freeze over the years. By the time they reach adulthood, their tissues lose about 15 percent of their moisture content, become less flexible, and become more susceptible to injury. Its muscle fibers begin to unite and develop cellular crosslinks that prevent parallel threads from moving independently. Slowly, our elastic fibers connect to the connective tissue of collagen and become increasingly inflexible. This healthy aging of tissues is eerily similar to the process of turning animal skins into leather. Unless we stretch, we dry and turn brown! Stretching slows down this drying process by stimulating the production of tissue lubricants. It separates the interlocking cell crosslinks and helps rebuild muscles with a healthy parallel cell structure.

Remember the cheap 70s sci-fi movie in which Raquel Welch and her team of miniaturized submarines are injected into someone's bloodstream? To truly understand how western physiology can benefit asana practice, we must create our internal odyssey and dive deep into the body to investigate how muscles work.

Flexibility and musculature
Muscles are organs: biological units made up of various specialized tissues that are integrated to perform a single function. (Physiologists divide the muscles into three types: the smooth muscles of the viscera; the specific cardiac muscles of the heart; and the striated muscles of the skeleton, but in this article, we will focus only on the skeletal muscles, which are known pulleys that we push towards the bones. body)

The specific function of muscles is, of course, the movement produced by muscle fibers, specialized cell bundles that change shape when contracting or relaxing. Muscle groups work together, alternate, and stretch in precise, coordinated arrangements to produce a full range of movements that our bodies are capable of.

In skeletal movements, the muscles that work (the muscles that contract to move the bones) are called "agonists." Different muscle groups, the muscles that need to be released and lengthened to allow movement, are called "antagonists." Almost all skeletal changes involve the coordinated action of agonist and antagonist muscle groups: they are the yang and yin of our movement anatomy.

But although stretching (lengthening antagonistic muscles) is half of the skeletal movement, most movement physiologists believe that increasing the elasticity of healthy muscle fibers is not an essential factor in improving flexibility. According to Michael Alter, author of Science of Flexibility (Human Kinetics, 1998), current research shows that individual muscle fibers can stretch to approximately 150 percent of their resting length before tearing. This stretch allows the muscles to move through a wide range of motion, enough for most stretching exercises, even the most difficult asanas.

What limits flexibility?
If your muscle fibers don't limit your stretching ability, what will? There are two primary science schools on what limits flexibility the most and what needs to be done to improve it. The first school focuses not on stretching the muscle fibers, but on increasing the elasticity of the connective tissues, encapsulating and connecting the cells that link the muscle fibers to other organs; the second deals with the "stretch reflex" and other functions of the autonomic (involuntary) nervous system. Yoga works on both. This is why it is such an effective method of increasing flexibility.

How long does it stretch to increase flexibility

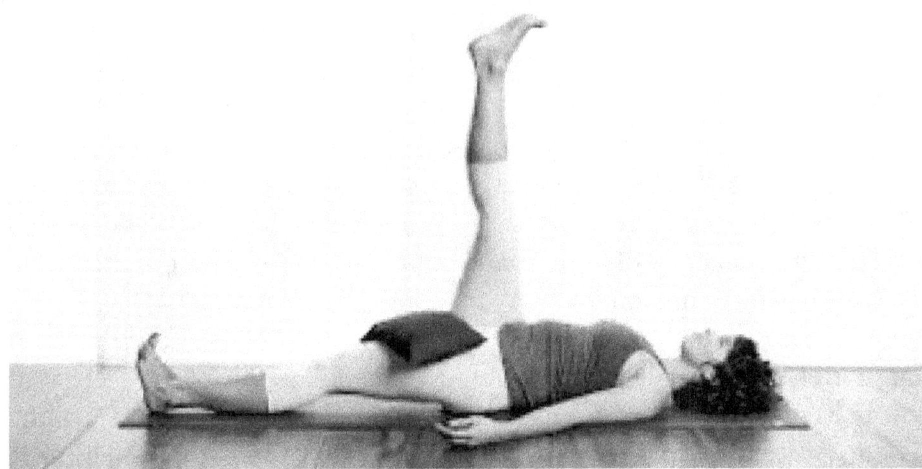

In these types of exercises, you maintain your posture long enough to affect the plastic quality of your connective tissue. Long stretching exercises like this can lead to permanent and healthy changes in the quality of the fascia that joins the muscles. Julie Gudmestad, a certified physical therapist and instructor at Iyengar, uses long-term asanas on patients at her clinic in Portland, Oregon. "If they hold the postures for shorter periods, people will have a good feeling of liberation," explains Gudmestad, "but they won't necessarily get the structural changes that lead to a permanent increase in flexibility."

According to Gudmestad, stretching exercises should be performed for 90 to 120 seconds to change the "soil substance" of the connective tissue. The ground powder is a gel-like, non-stringy cover fusing sinewy connective tissues, for example, collagen and elastin. Soil dust settles and greases up the connective tissue. Furthermore, it's, for the most part, accepted that impediments on this substance could restrain adaptability, particularly as we age.

By consolidating exact postural arrangement with the utilization of adornments, Gudmestad positions his patients to unwind in asanas so they can remain sufficiently long to roll out enduring improvements. "We ensure that individuals don't feel torment," says Gudmestad, "so they can inhale and extend longer."

How breathing helps increment adaptability

Kraftsow additionally stresses the significance of taking in a neurological work, taking note of that breath is a connection between our awareness and our autonomic sensory system. "It is this nature of breath," says Kraftsow, "that makes it an essential device in any study of self-advancement."

Pranayama, or breath control, is the fourth piece of a yogi's way to samadhi. One of the fundamental yoga rehearses enables the yogi to control the development of prana (essential vitality) all through the body. Be that as it may, regardless of whether saw through recondite yoga physiology or logical physiology in the West, the association between unwinding, extending, and breathing is entrenched. Physiologists portray this mechanical and neurological connection of development and breath, for instance, of synkinesis, the automatic construction of one piece of the body that happens with the difference in another part.

Yoga adaptability and reasoning.

Presently you might be pondering, "What do these western extending systems have to do with yoga?" On the one hand, extending is, obviously, a fundamental piece of building yoga deha, the yoga body with which the expert channels increasingly more prana. That is one reason why the colossal hatha yoga schools base their training on old-style asanas, a progression of stances that show and advance the entire scope of human development.

In any case, any great educator will likewise reveal to you that yoga isn't just about extending. "Yoga is an order that shows us better approaches to encounter the world," Judith Lasater, Ph.D., and a physical specialist, he clarifies, "with the goal that we can surrender our connection to our affliction." According to Lasater, there are just two asanas: cognizant or oblivious.

It is certainly possible to get so caught up in the pursuit of physical perfection that we lose sight of the "purpose" of asana practice: the state of samadhi. At the same time, however, exploring the limits of body flexibility can be a perfect way to develop concentration at one point necessary for the "inner limbs" of classical yoga.

Six ways to improve your flexibility

Do these simple movements in your routine to loosen up your muscles and maintain flexibility.
Flexibility is an essential part of physical fitness, which is often overlooked. Maintaining muscles is necessary to make daily activities effortless and feasible, to avoid injuries like back pain and for joints to function optimally and move through their more excellent range of motion.

1. yoga and improved flexibility
Yoga tops the list when it comes to versatility. Whatever your goal of flexibility, there is something for everyone when it comes to yoga. A style of yoga-like Yin or Hatha yoga can be an excellent first step if adaptability is your core interest.

Yin yoga works at an alternate pace with an accentuation on extending, breathing, and general unwinding. (See underneath for two of our preferred stances to attempt at home.)

2. Maintain your warm-up dynamics
Skipping warm-up is a no-no when it comes to staying flexible. Not only can you increase the risk of injury, but you will also miss a golden opportunity to improve flexibility. The inclusion of multi-muscle recruiting movements, such as multi-directional lunges, arm-length bridges, and a high knee jump, will help improve mobility both during and after your workout.

3. Vary your stretching exercises
Both static and dynamic extending have their place with regards to your adaptability. Static extending, where you hold the stretch, can help improve the scope of movement in a joint. However, it's ideal to leave it after exercise if your muscles are warm.
Before training, it is a good idea to include movement in your stretching exercises. Rotating lunges, pressing the knee against the circles of the chest and arm, Function admirably to improve adaptability as you set up the body for use.

4. Dancing works wonders for its flexibility
The comprehensive warm-up of dance classes not only provides a boost of flexibility but using muscles and joints in various ways through dance moves will also help extend them. Zumba is one of the most popular dance classes - all those shoulder and hip swirls, not to mention changes of direction, will do wonders for your flexibility.

5. Pilates is excellent for posture
While Pilates focuses on the core, movements like The Saw, Spine Stretch, and Neck Pull help improve flexibility everywhere, from the inner thighs and hips to the upper back and neck.

6. Realign the pelvis
There are a few reasons why an individual may encounter pelvic misalignment. Usually, changes in the pelvis occur due to an imbalance in the strength of the pelvic muscles, causing the muscles, joints, and bones of the pelvis to become misaligned.

Pelvic misalignment is one of the primary sources of back pain, hip and knee pain, as well as other musculoskeletal problems. There are several ways to realign the pelvis.

The pelvis is made of numerous bones that have melded. There is a group of bones on the left and a group on the right. These two groups of bones converge in the middle and are joined in the front by cartilage. If your pelvis is out of alignment, the entire base on which the muscles, nerves, and ligaments of the pelvic floor are located is disabled. There may be severe pelvic pain if it is misaligned. You may need medical treatments such as surgery or physical therapy to realign your pelvis. However, there are also specific exercises that can help you realign your pelvis at home.

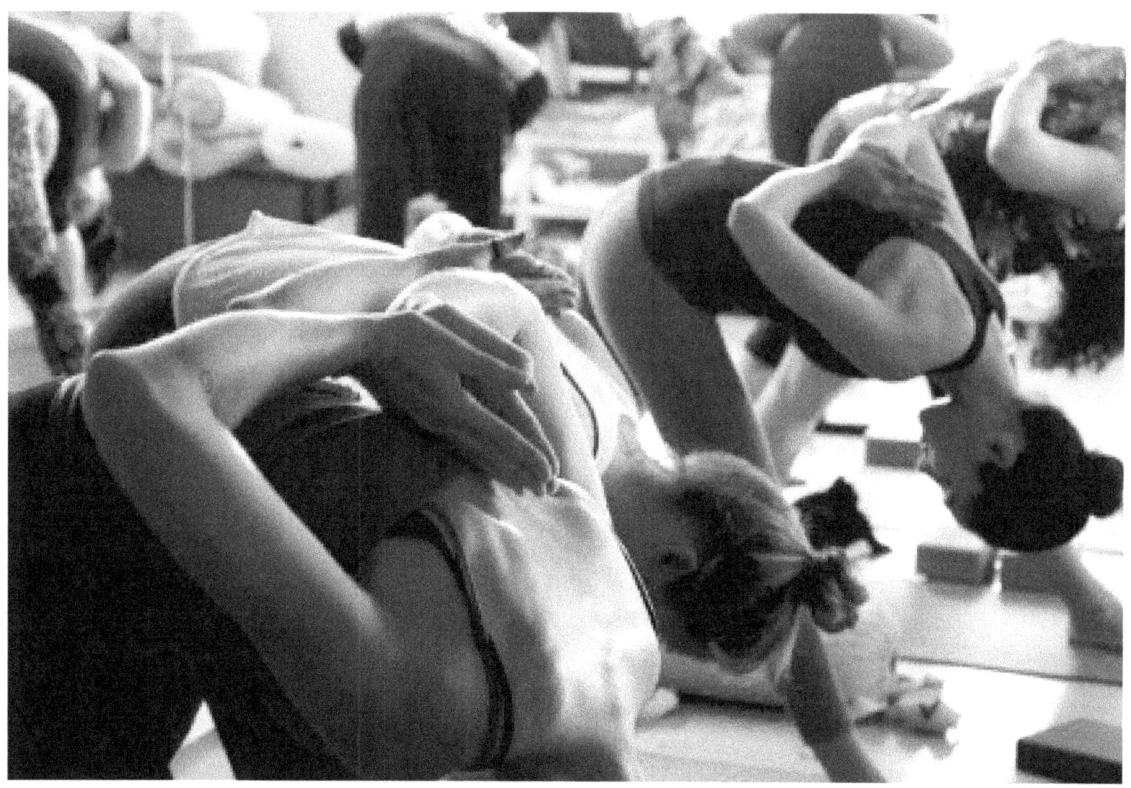

MAINTAIN OR IMPROVE RANGE OF MOTION
AND CIRCULATION

The scope of movement is the accessible measure of the development of a joint. Interestingly, adaptability is the capacity of delicate tissue structures, for example, muscle, ligament, and connective tissue, to extend through the available scope of joint movement. Regardless of whether it is experiencing remedial stretching during postinjury recovery or a standard adaptability program,

the connective tissue is the most basic physical focal point of scope of-movement works out. For ideal physiological possibilities to exist, the two scopes of movement and range of adaptability should be improved. The connective tissue associated with the body's reparative procedure after injury or medical procedure frequently restricts normal joint movement. In this way, understanding the biophysical elements of connective tissue is necessary for deciding ideal approaches to expand the scope of action because histological proof has demonstrated that fibrosis can happen inside four days of the beginning of fixed status. To successfully keep up and improve the scope of movement and adaptability,

information on both the related tissue structures and the different systems used to encourage the extensibility of these structures is necessary.

Range of motion
The scope of activity has been remembered for the audit of frameworks talked about before. Given the level of long haul dormancy and the absence of versatility seen in numerous people with ceaseless lung sickness, it is essential that the clinician test tolerant scope of movement at all significant joints. Shoulder support and thoracic spine scope of action are of specific significance in guaranteeing that chest extension aren't obstructed by delicate tissue snugness or absence of joint portability. Likewise, the lack of physical movement regular among individuals with incessant lung malady proposes that they keep up situated stances for significant stretches, which usually decreases flow in the lower limits.

Assessment of scope of movement utilizing exemplary goniometric systems,

inclinometer, and perception of useful degrees of an assortment of action is suitable. Additionally, the utilization of an essential measuring tape assists with learning thoracic extension in both the front back and transverse bearings. Chest calipers additionally called pelvimeters, help decide thoracic list and in recognizing changes in that file seen with dynamic endeavors at chest extension and with changes in hyperinflation

Increment Range Of Motion Through Exercises

Embracing a standard exercise routine will help increment your scope of movement. Your physical specialists ought to have a particular arrangement of activities intended to help improve your range of business, relying upon the joint and your present circumstance. The scope of movement is controlled by how far you can move a joint in every single, distinctive course. By dealing with specific activities that expand adaptability and manufacture quality, you ought to have the option to build your scope of movement.

Regardless of whether you are recuperating from a physical issue or don't have a custom exercise plan, constructing and keeping up your adaptability and scope of movement has numerous advantages. It can not just assist you with recuperating quicker from a physical issue, yet it can help keep future wounds from occurring in any case. Having better adaptability can likewise make ordinary every day exercises progressively pleasant, for example, twisting down to get something or getting in and out of your vehicle. When talking with your physical advisor about your activity schedule, make sure to consolidate practices that will expand adaptability and scope of movement...

REALIGN THE PELVIS

How to realign your pelvis?

To realign your pelvis, you have to extend tense or overactive muscles, fortify or actuate frail or hindered muscles, and train your cerebrum to keep your pelvis in the normal position.

Exercise can assist you with realigning your pelvis further. We will talk about the entire accepted procedures to realign your pelvis. Careful medications are fundamental in the treatment of severe instances of the skewed pelvis.

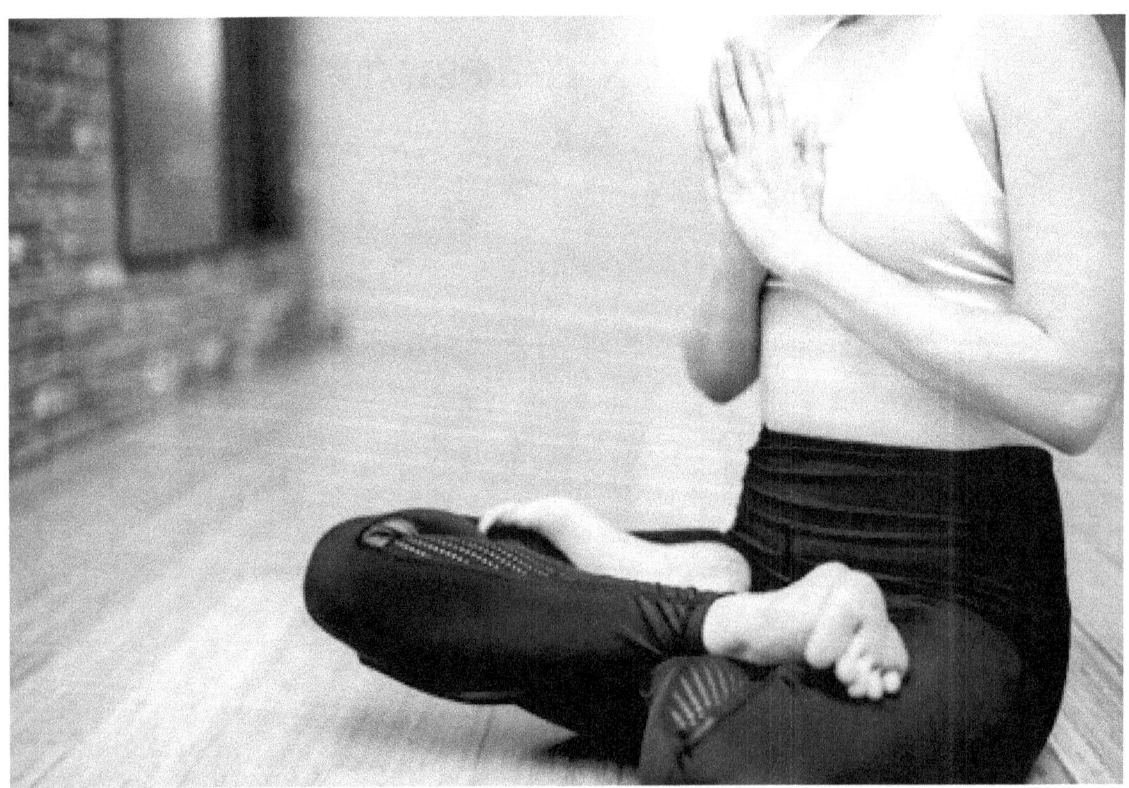

Below are some of the exercises to realign your pelvis.

Exercises to realign your pelvis:
Pelvic tilt exercise to realign your pelvis:
This exercise is useful for strengthening the pelvic muscles and helps correct pelvic misalignment. The steps to carry out this exercise are detailed below.

To begin the exercise, lie on the floor with your knees bent, feet flat on the floor, along with your head, shoulders, back, and arms.
Now slowly raise the hip by turning the pelvis, keeping in mind that only the lower back or bone should be lifted.
Hold this position for a few seconds. Be sure to maintain a normal breathing pattern here
Repeat this about 12 times a day
low-ab-workout-for-men-07

Realign the pelvis with abs:
Another exercise to realign your pelvis can be simple sit-ups. They are great for getting more muscular abs.

Lie down on the floor and try to curl up by lifting your upper body or head and shoulders off the floor.
Just try to lift your shoulders slightly off the floor, and don't force yourself to lift higher.
Repeat this ten times in one set.
You can do more than one or two sets of 10 repetitions each.
Full sit-up exercise
Knees to exercise the chest to realign the pelvis:
Another useful exercise to realign the pelvis or hips is the knee-to-chest exercise.

To begin the exercise, lie on your back. Bend your knees, so your feet stay flat on the floor, along with your head, shoulders, back, and hips.
Then try to bring one knee to your chest as much as possible.
Repeat the same with your other knee.
Perform four repetitions on each leg regularly.
Knee-to-Chest Stretches 1

Tables: a useful exercise to realign the pelvis:
Planks help you tone your abs and other muscle groups and keep your pelvis and hips in place as you develop your core strength.
Begin the exercise in a downward dog position with your arms shoulder-width apart
Now just stand on tiptoe and forearms, support your body up, off the floor.
Hold this position as long as possible. You can extend the time, holding the table to about 60 seconds.
You can also opt for side planks or one-leg planks to add variety to the movement.

Realign the pelvis with a seated lateral stretch:
This exercise helps stretch the hip abductor muscles, helping to realign the pelvis.

To begin the training, sit on the floor and straighten both legs.
Then hold your right foot with your right hand and raise your left hand above your head while leaning towards you as far as possible.
Hold this for a couple of moments and afterward come back to the beginning position.
Rehash a similar stretch with the opposite side.
Complete four reps on each side and do 8 of those pieces a day.

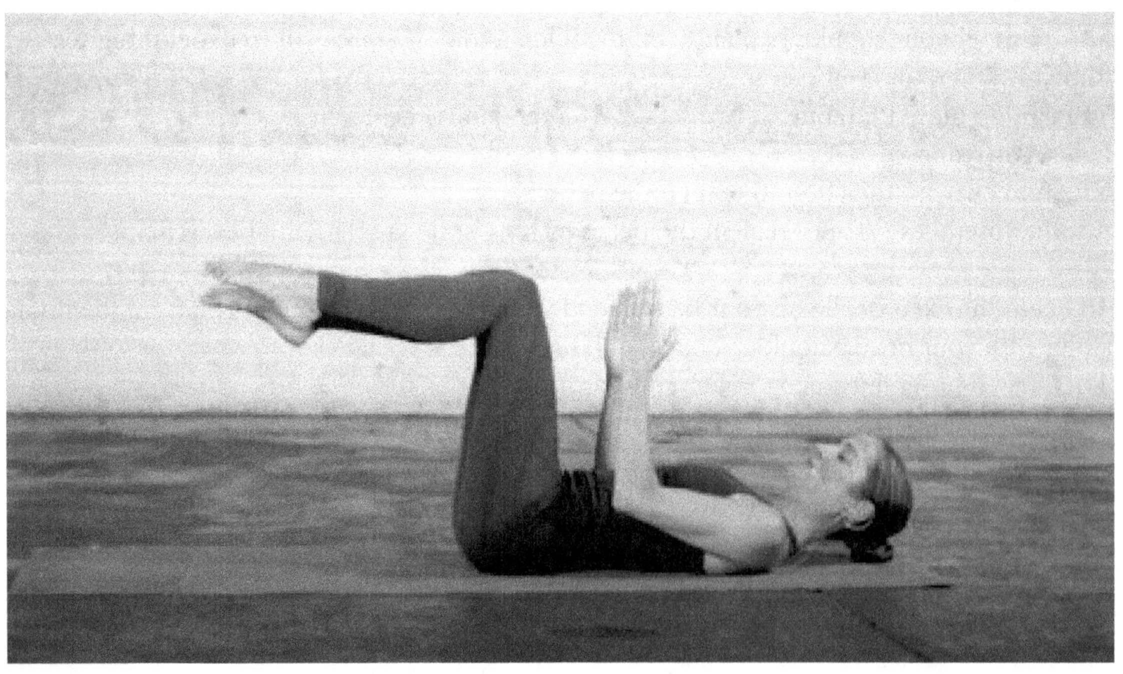

Prone hip extensions:
This exercise helps strengthen the lower back and leg muscles on the weaker side. However, it should be noted that pregnant hips should not bend.

- Hold a pad under your hips and lie on your stomach.
- Curve your knee on the more vulnerable side while lifting your lower leg
- Somewhat lift your thigh while keeping your knee twisted at a 90-degree edge.
- Gradually lower your leg and come back to the beginning position. Perform 8 of such reiterations; 3 times each week.

Side hip additions:
- This is a lower back and leg stretch that helps realign the pelvis.
- Lie on your side (left) on the floor and bend your left arm to rest your head on the palm of your hand. Keep your right arm on the story to support your body.
- Slowly raise your right leg at a 45-degree angle.
- Lower your leg and rest for about 2 seconds, then repeat.
- Do eight repetitions and repeat the same on the other side 2-3 times a week.
- Eventually, you can increase it to about 12 repetitions.

Iliotibial band stretch to realign the pelvis:
The iliotibial band is the connective tissue that extends from the knee down the side of the leg to the external pelvis.
Here it may be necessary to stretch the iliotibial band. Keep in mind that pregnant women should avoid this exercise.

- First, stand on your side next to a wall
- Then move one of your legs away from the wall behind the other leg.
- Then lean the side of your hip with your leg crossed to the wall to feel a stretch.
- Hold the position for about 30 seconds.
- Rest a few seconds and do the same thing four times.
- Then do the same thing four more times with the other side.

STRENGTHEN WEAK MUSCLES

Regular yoga is practiced to strengthen the internal and external muscles, but YIN yoga is practiced to strengthen the joints of the body. You can say that it is the practice of balance for the yang style of yoga. The main difference between yin yoga and other forms of yoga is that yin yoga is not restorative yoga. So, if you damage some tissues of your body and try to repair it by practicing yin yoga, think again, because in that case, yin yoga will be more harmful than beneficial. The purpose of yin yoga is similar to any other style of yoga. The stimulation typically created in the asana position is practiced very deeply compared to muscle or superficial tissues (which we call yang tissues). The purpose of yin yoga is to connect tissues such as bones, ligaments, and joints of the body that are not commonly practiced when various other styles of yoga asanas are practiced.

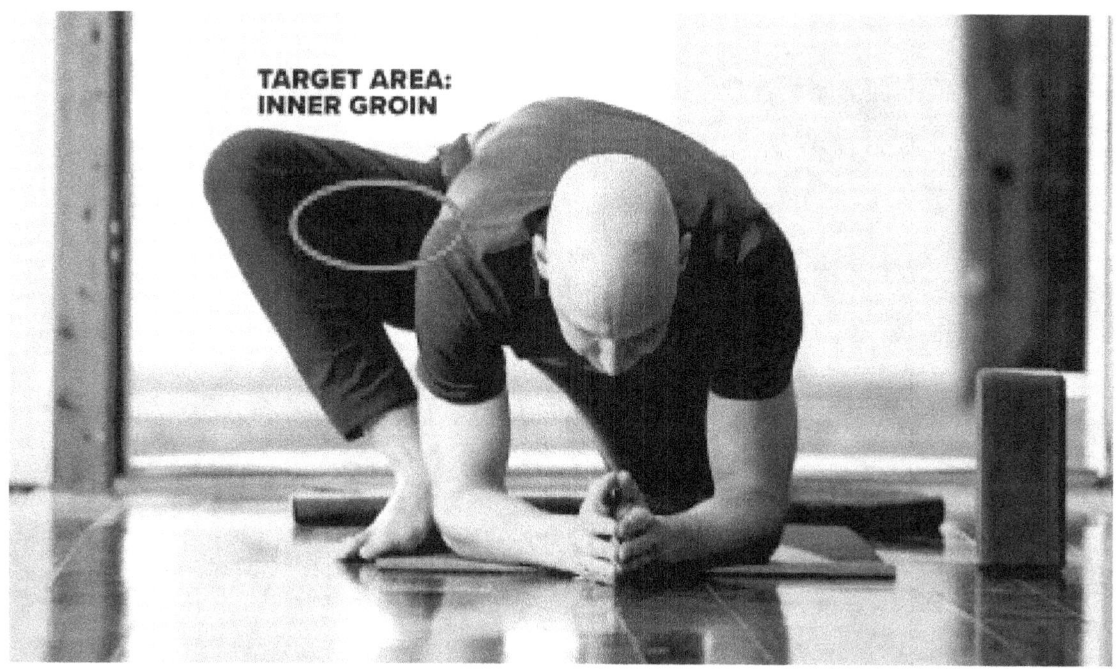

Anahatasana (heart melting)

To enter the pose, you must sit on all fours. Move your hands forward so that your chest rests on the floor, and your hips are just above your knees. You should try to keep your hands broad across your shoulder. The advantage of this pose is open shoulders, a gentle curve for the upper and middle back. To get out of this position, you can slide forward on your stomach or return to the child's place. The joints affected by this posture are the shoulder/humerus joint, slight stress on the lower back, and provides excellent compression on the upper back.

Ankle stretch

To adopt the pose, you must sit on your heels. If your knees or ankle develop excruciating pain, this pose is not right for you. It is excellent retention for squats or finger exercises. It is a potent stimulant for four meridians that flow through the feet and ankles, opening and strengthening the ankles. Initially, you need to hold this position for one minute, and gradually, the waiting period can be extended according to your tolerance limit. The areas that benefit from this pose are the spleen, liver, stomach, and gallbladder lines, while the affected joint is the ankle joint.

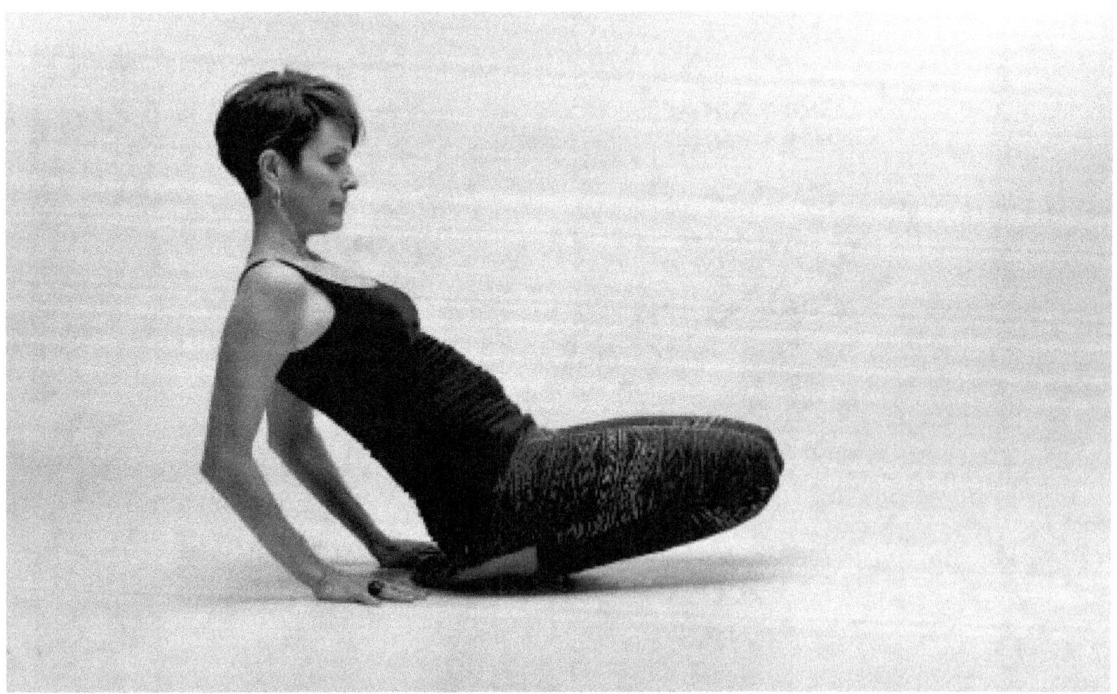

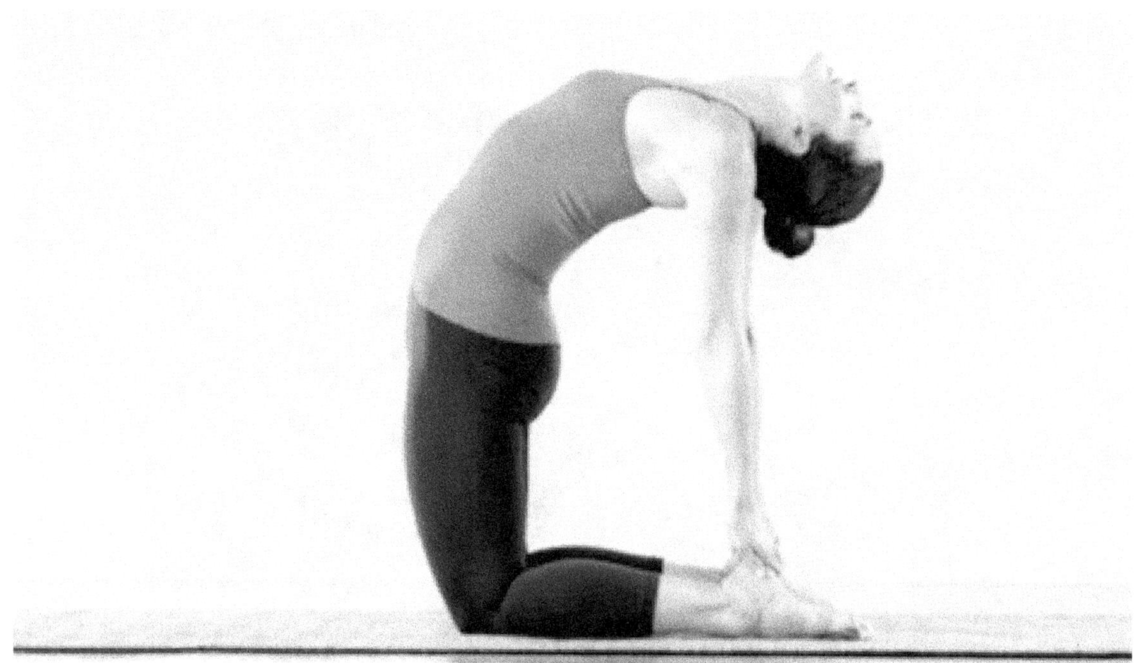

Camel pose

A safe way to adopt this pose is to sit on your heels, as in the case of ankle stretching, Thighs and your forehead are on the floor, and lift your hips forward. When the hips move forward, the back arches. Then you have to lower your head back. If you have neck problems, try to keep your chin against your chest. This pose is suitable for those with dropped shoulders or arched backs as it opens the shoulders, stretches the hip flexors, intensely flexes the sacral/lumbar spine and opens the upper thighs, and provides openings at the ankles. The ankles, shoulders, and back joints benefit from this posture.

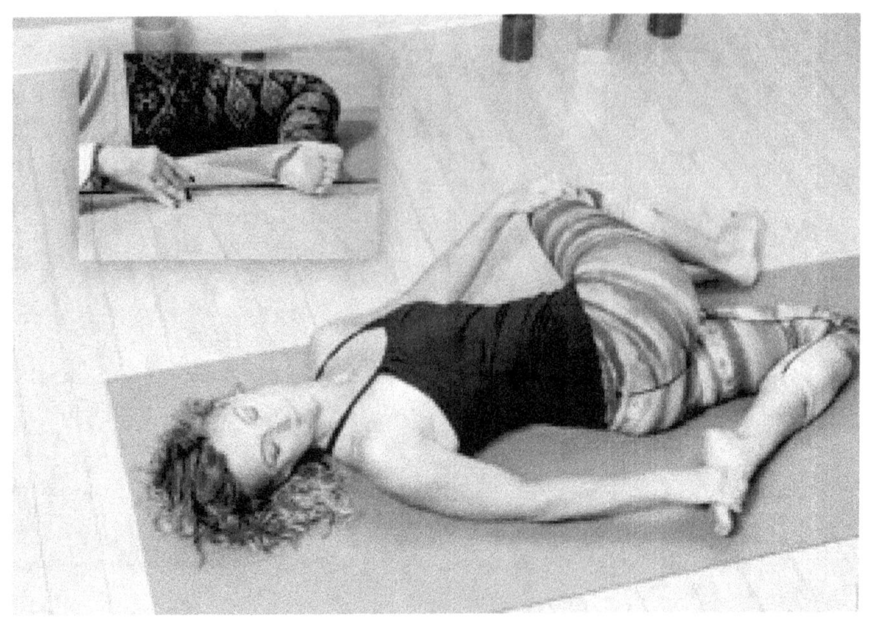

Cat pulls his tail

To start in this pose, you must sit with both legs facing you. Then when you turn right, you should lie on your right elbow. Keep your right leg straight and bring your left leg forward and sideways. Bend your right leg so that your heels are closer to your glutes. Now grab with your left hand to grab your right foot. Now try to get your foot away from you. This pose opens your thighs and quads, slightly compresses your lower back, and is a good hold for very sharp forward bends.

Child pose

This pose requires sitting on your heels and then slowly bending forward so that your chest rests on your thighs and your forehead are on the floor. This pose is beneficial for the spine and ankle as it provides relief from back pain and neck pain. Gently compresses the stomach and chest and is useful for digestion. The child's posture is a healing and calming attitude.

Hanging

In this pose, you should be at hip-width with both feet. Leaning forward, hold your elbows with your opposite hands. This pose gently extends through the lower spine, warms the quads and loosens the hamstrings, compresses the stomach and internal organs, develops strength in the diaphragm, massages the abdominal organs, and heals menstrual cramps. The joints of the back are mainly affected by this posture. This pose is perfect for the liver, kidneys, and spleen. This posture strongly stimulates the urinary bladder meridian due to intense stretching along the back of the spine and legs.

Toe Squat

You should sit on your toes and keep your feet together. Be on the balls of your feet. This pose strengthens the ankles and opens the feet and toes, stimulating the six meridian lines of the lower body. Here the ankles and toes benefit from this pose. All the lower body meridians are stimulated by compression on the toes. The front of the ankles is also compressed, which helps open the lines of the liver, spleen, stomach, and gallbladder.

INCREASE ENERGY LEVEL

There's no doubt that long hours of traffic, desk-related chores, and endless chores lead to complete mental and physical exhaustion. Due to the overworked body, many people are unable to do their hobbies or find it difficult to do any other form of exercise. This is all due to low energy levels and insufficient prana (life force) in the body. The impeccable, daily practice of yoga provides the much-needed energy boost that provides practitioners with energy for the rest of the day. Yoga practices are very effective in reducing body and mental fatigue, increasing energy levels in the body. Yoga is also best known for reducing stress levels, which ultimately increase energy levels in the body.

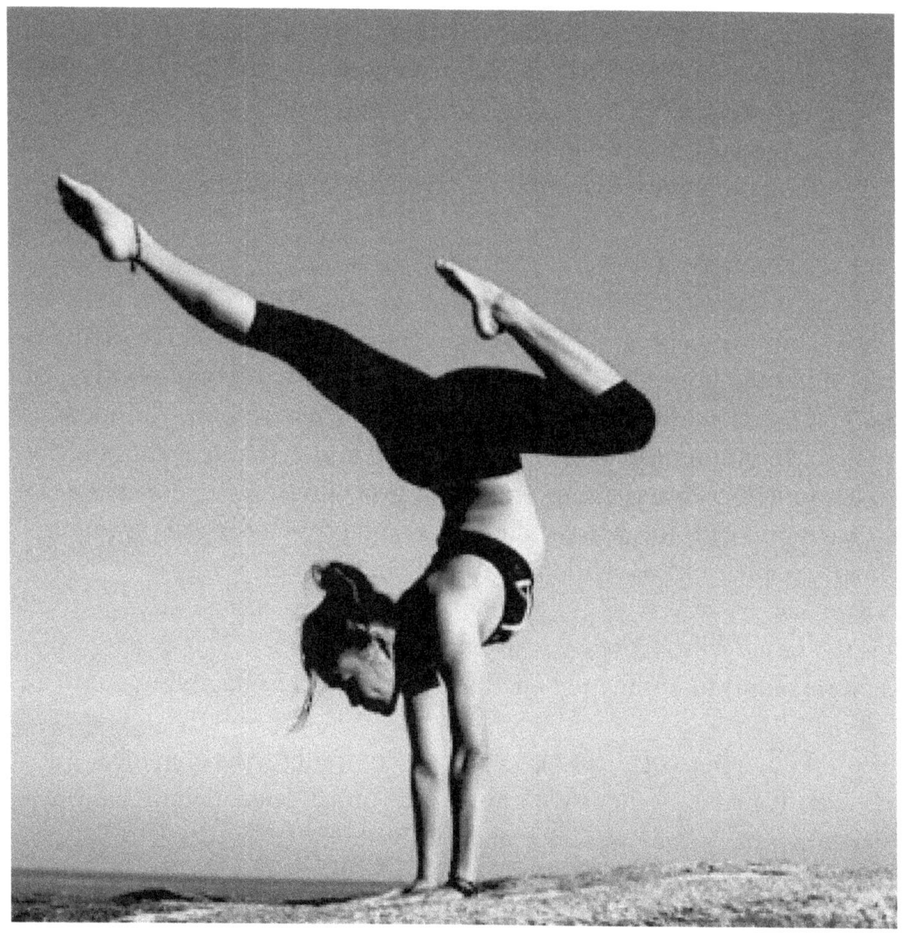

Energize your core with yoga practices, clean eating, and a good night's sleep. Wake up to a beautiful morning with strength and vitality. Here is a list of three great ways yoga increases your energy. Check out the tips below:

1. Yoga Poses: Probably, no one can think of practicing yoga without performing yoga poses regularly. Yoga asanas are the most cost-effective way to relax and rejuvenate the body and mind. Some entities can avoid moving the body in different directions and shapes. Still, the fact is that performing yoga poses removes blockages along the spinal cord and smooths the flow of energy in the body.

2. Yogic Breathing Techniques: Don't be surprised if you learn that changing your breathing patterns can make a significant difference in your health and energy levels. Most people breathe very shallowly in their daily lives, resulting in less oxygen supply to the body's organs. Conscious breathing ensures optimal oxygen exchange with the rest of the body, leading to increased energy and a healthier body system. Practice different breathing techniques such as pranayama with a shiny skull, three-piece yoga breathing, alternate nose breathing technique, etc., which regulate blood flow in the body, calm the mind, and stimulate the senses. Yoga deep breathing exercises are potent in activating the Kundalini energy.. These seven chakras are considered to be the body's energy centers that, when stimulated, resulting in increased awareness, creativity, and harmony.

3. Meditation: Different people want extra vitality and diligence to get through the day. To meet demand, many of us rely on substances like energy drinks, vitamins, etc., which only provide a temporary energy boost. For permanent results, include meditation practices. Meditation has the power to suppress negative feelings and gain positive experiences. Peaceful meditation dramatically improves the body's stress response and leads to increased energy flow. Meditation exercises calm the mind and promote feelings of love, peace, and eternal happiness. When the mind rests in a peaceful state, a person can live in the present and harmony with the self. Meditation also increases the cosmic energy in the body that helps people to have vivid and vibrant experiences.

How yoga is the best way to increase your energy level
- Everyone seems to know the benefits of yoga, such as flexibility, calm, and concentration.
- Did you know that yoga can also increase your energy level in life?
- Practicing yoga strengthens your ability to control your mental and physical being, so yoga also dramatically increases your energy level.

- Each pose or asana affects a different set of muscles in your body. Therefore, yoga is the best way to energize your mind, body, and soul for the challenges of everyday life.
- You breathe slowly, which helps you calm down and improves your mental ability to maintain postures.
- Each pose increases connectivity with the mind and body by breaking the connection with the external environment.

Yoga and cortisol balance
- Cortisol is broadly known as a pressure hormone, which we, as a whole, need to decrease to feel positive and energized. Too much cortisol builds tension and stress, which can prompt gloom and uneasiness regularly.
- But simultaneously, you likewise can't have too little cortisol part in your framework.
- Too low levels of cortisol and your body cause problems like fatigue, low blood pressure, gastrointestinal, and reproductive problems.
Here comes the beauty of practicing yoga regularly. Its cortisol level achieves optimal balance, giving you a sustainable feeling of energy in life.

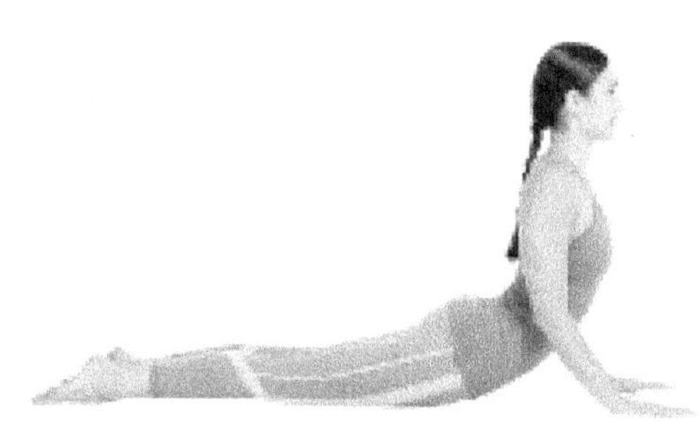

Yoga and stress relief
•	Stress is generally associated with the mind. But your mind and body play an important role in determining your stress levels.
•	For example, focusing on one thing for hours, like a computer screen, creates a stressful mood. That stress comes from your mind, as does the muscle tension in your neck, lower back, and other parts of your body.
•	Thanks to yoga, you can reduce stress both physically and mentally. You give in to various postures that can help your muscles minimize stress.
•	At the same time, you breathe deeply and become aware of your breathing.
•	Breathing profoundly relaxes and focuses your mind. Your overall immune system improves to increase your energy level.
•	Deep breathing is the most basic form of yoga, and you can do it anywhere - at home, at your desk, or even on the go.
•	When in a stressful situation, deep breathing naturally reduces stress levels.
Yoga and blood flow
•	Different yoga poses and deep breathing send more oxygen to the blood flow in your body. Increased oxygen improves circulation and blood flow.
•	This means that you get an optimal amount of blood flow in your brain and other parts of your body.
•	As a result, his mind feels alert, and his reflex instincts also increase. Your overall body function improves through improved blood flow.
•	Blood flow and oxygen levels decrease if you spend most of the day sitting.
•	Regular yoga breaks the cycle of an energy-efficient lifestyle. Her spine is significantly stretched, which strengthens the neural network that connects her body to her mind.

Yoga and sleep quality
Sleep duration is not as important as sleep quality, which is why most people feel tired even after 7 to 8 hours of sleep.
When your mind and body are stressed, it affects your ability to hit brain waves, helping you get a good night's sleep. This is when yoga becomes a great help.
With regular yoga exercises, you can remove stress from your body and mind. And that helps you sleep well every night. The next morning always brings a little energy, and you feel active all day.

ELEVATE MOOD AND RELIEVE SADNESS AND DEPRESSION

Many yoga poses can do wonders for your mind and body. From hundreds of such posts, I have selected the top three yoga poses, particularly useful for depression and anxiety. The first, called Salute to the Sun, is not one pose but a succession of twelve poses. You should always lie on your back for a few minutes and breathe easily to finish your mental health yoga session every day. Yoga for uneasiness and sadness should be possible once, twice, or three times each day, contingent upon your available time and enthusiasm..

A yoga session can last from twenty minutes to an hour; a regular course is thirty minutes. Forty-five minutes usually is quite a while to do all the yoga models for tension and gloom with feeling and focus. Yoga poses should not be confused with merely stretching the limbs. Every pore in your existence speaks to you when you do it with passion, and yoga for mental health offers the best results.

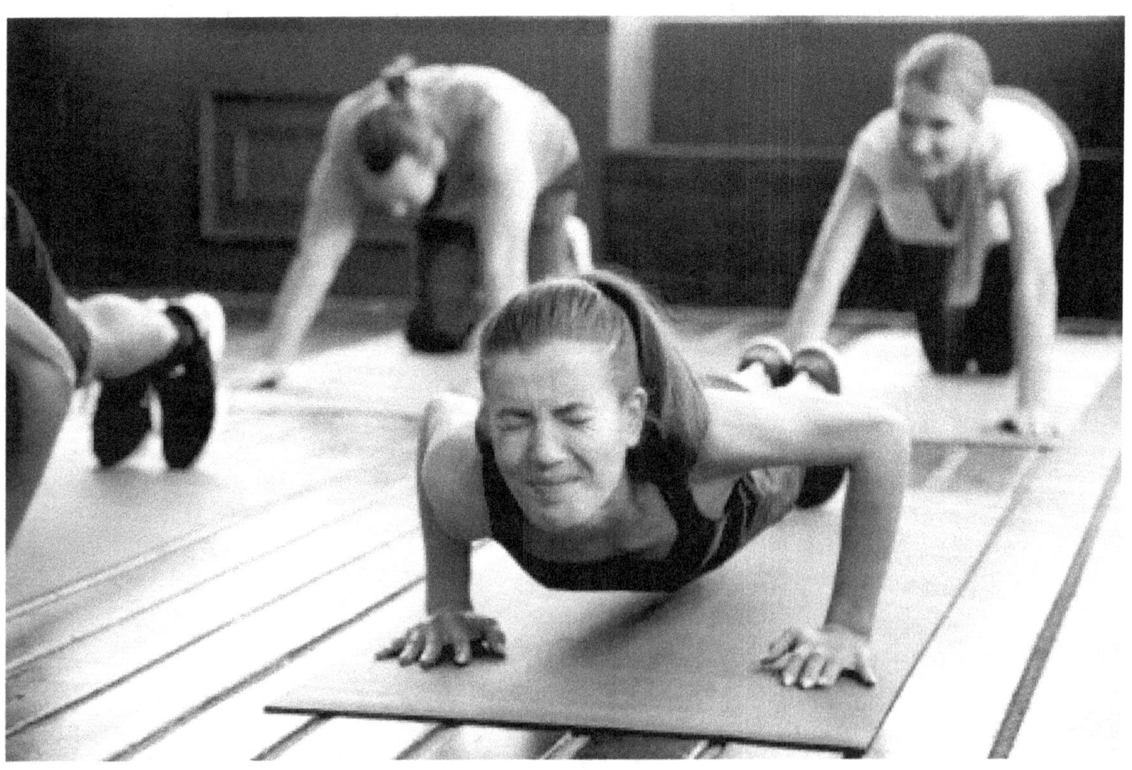

1. The greeting to the sun
Yoga exercises and consists of a series of twelve yoga postures with an emphasis on
inhalation and exhalation with each step of the salute. It seems simple enough, but it is a
beneficial yoga for depression and anxiety. It spreads throughout the body and channels
the flow of different energies. Here's how to do it:

First position
Take a deep breath. Stand up straight, body relaxed but straight. Put your hands together
and join them to your heart in the Namaste pose. Exhale

Second position
Begin inhaling and gently spread your hands and raise them above your head, fully extending your arms. Fold back with your palm toward the air. Do not bend more than you can
comfortably.

Third place
Now exhale slowly and lean forward with your legs stretched out. Your brow is corresponding to the ground yet doesn't contact it. Hold your breath. You should touch the floor
with your hands. If you can't bend to hit the ground, bend as much as you can.

Fourth position
Stretch your left leg back, with your knee and toe contacting the floor. Present your correct pin with your knee nearly to your chest and foot, entirely and solidly on the floor. Lift
your jaw and inhale delicately and profoundly.

Fifth position
Bring your left leg back halfway and stretch your right leg halfway, so they are comparing
to each other.Lift your hips as though you are going to push up. Your body now forms a
table. Keep your chin against the esophagus. Begin to exhale gently and move on to the
next yoga position for euphoria and depression as you exhale.

Sixth position
Stretch your legs back and get down. Her palms, chest, knees, and toes touch the floor.
Her hips stay slightly raised, and her belly doesn't touch the ground at all. This denotes
the finish of the sun greeting, a yoga pose that is viable for wretchedness and tension.

Seventh position
Begin to breathe gently. Extend your arms, lower your legs and waist so that your toes,
legs, knees, thighs, and groin touch the floor and gently lift your torso.

Lift your chin as if you are looking up and stretching your neck.

Eighth position
Raise your hips and bring your legs straight halfway. Your body now forms the same triangle. Lower your head and close your chin toward your esophagus and exhale gently. His palms and heels remain flat and firmly planted on the ground.

Ninth position
Breathe gently, stretch your right leg back, bend your spine, and bring your left leg forward with your knee against your chest. The toe and knee of the right leg touch the floor, and the left foot is flat on the floor. Your palms are flat on the ground. Lift your chin. You are now in the same yoga posture to reduce stress and anxiety as in the fourth position, but with the straight alternative leg.

Tenth position
Unite your feet, fix your legs, and twist forward from the midriff. Presently your stance is equivalent to in the third position.. Try to touch the floor again with your palms, and if you can't, lower them as much as possible. Gently breathe out and release stress and anxiety.

Eleventh position
Breathe deeply and gently. Stretch your body and bend backward with your palms up. This is the same position as in the second position.

Twelfth position
Stretch your body out with your palms facing each other (as if taking the Namaste pose) and exhale gently. Hold every yoga pose for a couple of moments. This is near. In the second round, substitute your legs: first, stretch your correct leg in the fourth position and your left leg in ninth.
There is a variety of this yoga act for uneasiness and sorrow in which a similar leg is extended in the fourth and ninth positions and substitutes just in the following round. It is recommended to lie on your back for a few minutes in the corpse pose (Shavasana) after completing your anxiety yoga session at sun salutation.
The ancient method also includes chanting the seed syllables of the Sun Mantra while making the Sun Salutation. Texts that explain solar science believe that the rays of the first minutes at dawn are therapeutic and healing and support yoga for mental health. Ideally, the sun salutation is done in the direction of the sun at sunrise.
In case you experience the evil impacts of distress and anxiety, you will on a fundamental level benefit by doing these yoga presents. The first is known as a shoulder support.

It is known as Sarvanga asana in Sanskrit. Sarvanga suggests all the organs or parts. This yoga represents disquiet, and melancholy conveys vitality to the whole body and mind. Your center and legs reached out to the most outrageous as you stand up vertically, with your neck twisted and your head laying on the floor, while the heaviness of your whole body puts on your shoulders. You hold your body with your hands. Here are the means to do it:

Lie on your back. Loose, however, straight. Keep your legs together, with your lower legs contacting and your fingers facing up. Keep your arms straight and your palms stroking your thighs.

Delicately breathe in as you gradually raise your legs and completely stretch them at a ninety-degree edge. Breathe out and lift your body as you breathe in. Carry your hands to your midsection to help your chest area as you rise. Raise your body as straight as could be expected under the circumstances. Keep your legs together this time. The whole weight of your body should lay on your shoulders (not on your neck or head). Your jaw contacts the throat. Your toes should now highlight the roof. Inhale tranquility and normally. Stay right now for thirty seconds for uneasiness and misery. You can slowly build the term, yet ought not to surpass three minutes.

To finish the asana, tenderly curve your legs, go them to your knees, and gradually bring down your body, utilizing your hands to help the weight. When the body is back on the floor, fix your legs, and relax. This position is brilliant for the spine, sensory system, and thyroid. Toward the finish of your yoga meeting for misery and nervousness, consistently rests in the body present for three to five minutes.

3. The child poses

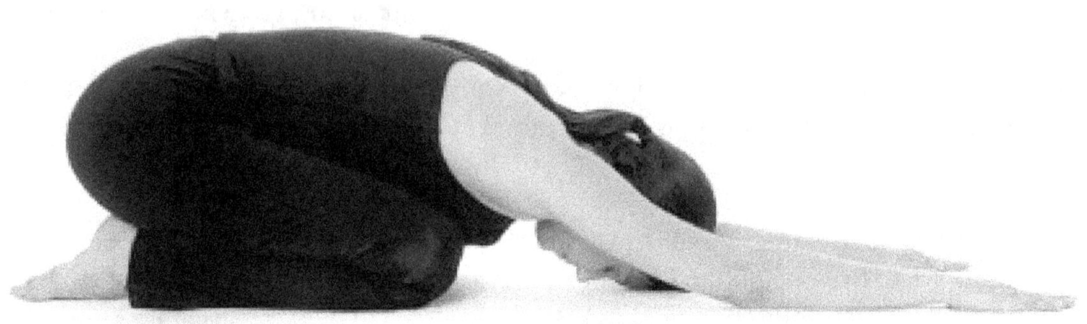

It is called Bala Asana. Bala means boy. It is a simple and easy yoga pose for anxiety that has a calming effect on the body and mind. Follow the steps below to perform the pose: Keep your legs hip-width apart and inhale gently as you kneel on your hands and knees. Your headrests in your arms and your palms down. Stretch your toes so that your toenails touch the floor, so they stay relaxed. This naturally stretches the torso and folds the neck when folded over the thighs so that the forehead touches the floor. Breathe gently and bring your arms along your legs. The palms will now point up. Breathe slowly and hold this fear yoga pose for thirty seconds. To complete this yoga pose for anxiety and depression, bring your arms forward with your palms down, bring your torso forward, and get up.

You can place a pillow between the buttocks and heels if the stretch is not pleasant Don't hesitate to lay your brow on a pad if the floor feels hard or awkward.

Regulation of breathing.

There is a term that is often found in most yogic scriptures.

It is called Pranayama. Prana means vital force in the breath, and Yama means to lengthen, strengthen, or advance. Pranayama is the science of regulating breathing, which has powerful effects on reducing anxiety, depression, and stress. It is mainly made up of twelve different types. It has three phases, called exhalation (rechaka), retention (kumbhaka), and inhalation (puraka). Pranayama is not for everyone: correct regulation of breathing requires perfect silence in posture and strict nutritional and moral behavior. But, above all, because through pranayama, you provide the vital force of each pore of your body. If your mood is negative and your breath is impure, this is what will push and deliver all cells.

Each cell is a complete housing unit in itself. It has a respiratory framework, an excretory framework, a sensory system, and an endocrine framework. The quality of the life force it provides to each cell affects the life and health of that cell. Pranayama can open blocked blood vessels, make muscles flexible, brighten skin, reduce stiffness in joints, and bring veins to life. However, improperly done pranayama can lead to neurological disorders. That being said, if you can't hold your breath during pranayama, don't worry if you practice depression and anxiety along with yoga.

At the point when you breathe in and breathe out with a specific goal in mind, it manages your breathing. It quickly gives your psyche harmony, assisting with decreasing uneasiness and negative considerations related to sadness. Of the numerous sorts, I will impart to both of you kinds of pranayama that are especially useful in treating sadness and tension with yoga.

Before beginning pranayama, it is fundamental to sit with your back straight, with your back, neck, and head in a straight line. If you can relax with folded legs, it is far better since it controls the vital energies in the body. You can likewise unwind in a seat. In any event, two hours must pass between your supper and the pranayama work out. On the off chance that you do yoga and, at that point, do pranayama, the compensations of that yoga for diminishing uneasiness and wretchedness are progressively huge and quicker all things considered.

alternative breathing

Alternative Breathing is a type of pranayama that is excellent for neurological and re-spiratory cleansing and detoxification, and a great addition to yoga for depression and anxiety. It is part of the nervous system regime (Nadi-shodhana).Breathing (kumbhaka) is an essential aspect of pranayama for depression and anxiety.

Such breathing in the real sense of the word is recommended for those who master physi-cal posture and are only on a sattvic diet and abstain entirely. Furthermore, it is a gradual progress. Therefore, in a variety of standard alternative breathing.

There is a fundamental reason to take this seriously. When you breathe alternately wi-thout gaining a stable posture and without controlling your diet, you risk pushing toxins through your nervous system to all parts of the body. This can lead to neurological disor-ders, tumor formation, cysts, and memory loss. However, practicing it without prolonged breathing gives you the most significant benefit of pranayama and yoga for depression and anxiety. It purifies and cleanses your nervous system and stimulates You are settling energies and powers in and around you. In any case, do not go beyond what is comfor-table for you. Yoga exercises aren't supposed to make you look red, during, or after. They should be effortless.

RELEASE NEGATIVE OR STAGNANT ENERGY AND EMOTIONS

One of the beautiful gifts that yoga offers us is the opportunity to sit down with uncomfortable emotions and continue working with them. This is especially true for me when I develop a Yin yoga practice. Being trapped for 5-10 minutes not only releases the body physically, but we also find mental and emotional release. For people going through things from their past or current situations, this can be incredibly powerful and healing. It can also be excruciating to bring up these emotions, so I want to warn people to have other supports in creating space to allow painful feelings to arise.

In general, the following poses are great for helping you find a release, physical, mental, and emotional.

Hip openers

Vast numbers of us will, in general, store our feelings in the hip area. This is an essential piece of the "battle or flight" stress reaction. Every time we feel threatened or have a stress response, we respond physically by tensing ourselves in this area or pulling or fleeing to protect ourselves.

But even after the threat has passed, there is still an emotional scar from what triggered the situation. When we do not process these emotions, they remain stagnant and prevent us from moving forward.

The space between the hips is likewise the area of the second chakra or vitality focus. This chakra is connected to our associations with others, which are regularly the wellspring of troublesome feelings, be it deserting, hatred, or misfortune. At the point when the chakra is shut or uneven, you may see troubles in your connections and the sentiment of being trapped.Igniting this hip-opening chakra is a way to open yourself up to processing, find forgiveness, and understand the root of your emotions.

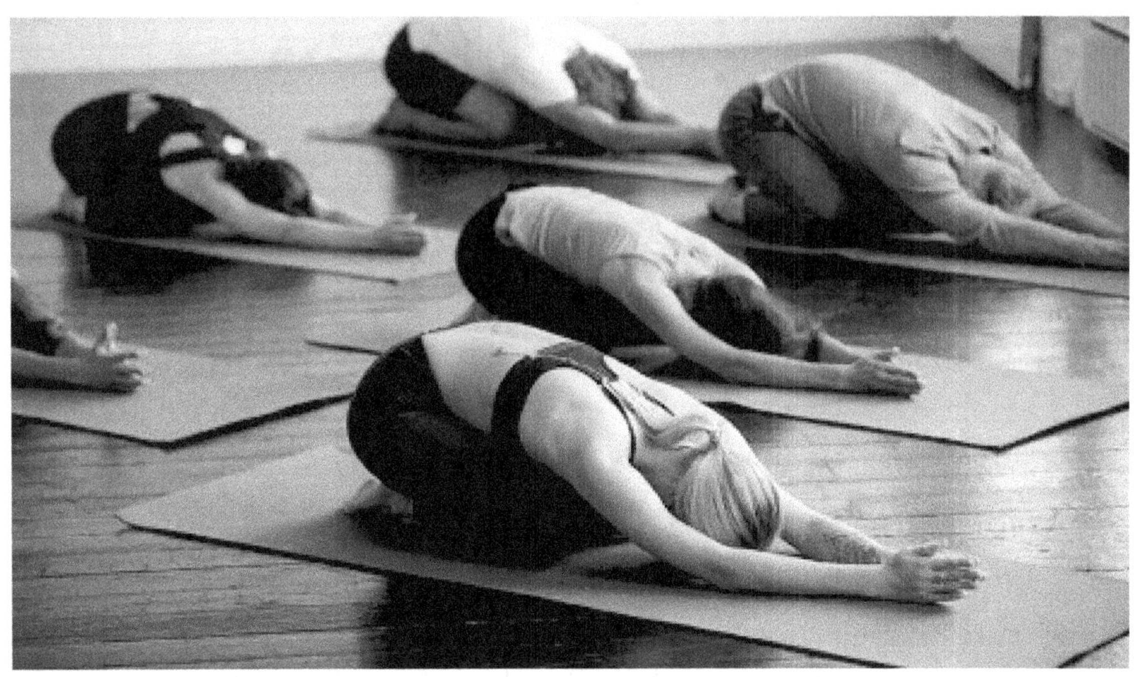

1. recline angle

You can rehearse this posture with or without embellishments. Having a pad under the spine makes it a heart opener just as a hip opener, which will expand the sentiment of discharge. I likewise prefer to rehearse this posture with one hand on my heart and the other on the space between my hips.

2. Pigeon pose

Pigeon is one of the most profound hip openers we practice in yoga, and regularly one of the most physical and mental difficulties. Utilize all the extras you need to feel bolstered and rest a little in the posture. Exploit that sentiment of help as a chance to celebrate and investigate unhesitatingly to let everything come to do that

.3. Child's attitude

Take this pose with your knees wide to create a hip opening. This posture is called so precise because it allows us to snuggle up and embrace a child's virtues. When we grow up, we allow ourselves to become vulnerable.

In this way, we can be used to it, without the need to impress, act, or react in any particular way. It is an invitation to withdraw to childhood and let our emotions flow freely as before.

Twists

Turns are convincing for processing and vigorously preparing things. As indicated by Ayurveda, the sister study of yoga, sound processing is fundamental; for the nourishment, we eat as well as for the encounters we gain.

These encounters can incorporate discussions with individuals, the earth around us, our reactions to things, all of which bring out our feelings. Rehearsing turns invigorates the stomach related framework and supports the activity of handling.

4. Turn supported

Use one large pillow or two smaller pillows and a blanket to create a beautiful, supportive bed. Bring one hip to the side of the pad and twist, bending your torso down. Bring both cheeks to the cushion. Focus on your breathing, and watch what happens. Actively relax all parts of the body and allow yourself to relax.

Relaxing poses where the body does not do much physically, except existing ones, are perhaps the most powerful. When the body is silent, the mind often wanders. Use this space to return thoughts to body and mind. Take an inventory of how the frame and state of mind feel.

If something becomes unbalanced, you start to become curious about why and what is the source of this feeling. Direct your attention to that discomfort and, instead of pushing it down, create the space to invite it.

5. Legs against the wall

This pose is such a sweet release; it purifies the energy in the body. We physically allow the legs to dissipate the old heat and mentally melt away the heaviness.

There are various varieties of this posture. You can begin altogether without frill, or attempt it with specific backings under the hips and the spine. You can likewise put a square on your feet for a little weight and a cover over your body for warmth and security.

6. Savasana

In such a rush in our lives to each other, we always do ourselves an invaluable favor when we can find complete silence. The mind needs these moments of silence to process and reflect. You have to remove the stimuli to understand all the things you need every day.

Instead of mentally spending your Savasana on your shopping list, try your best to be on your mind and body, it may be your only chance to do it all day. Silently watch what appears and be open to any significant changes that may occur.

Often we don't understand the cause of our emotions. We are not sure why we are angry, sad, or depressed. It may be that there is a profound and deep-rooted answer that we need time and space to understand. But making friends with your mind and body is one way to bring these things to the surface. Opening the parts of the body that contain these emotions is another piece of the puzzle. Try practicing these poses; They can lead you to a breakthrough that will give you some clarity and help you overcome your difficult emotions.

How to relieve aches and pains with yoga
Some of yoga's most obvious benefits include an incredibly taut body, more flexibility, and better balance. One of the other great benefits that are often overlooked is that it can also ease aches and pains.
Yoga can provide relief from a variety of different pains and conditions, including
Joint pain Headache Digestive problems Muscle pain or stiffness Back pain Knee pain Many other joint chronic pains
Keep in mind that improving flexibility is generally the best way to relieve most aches and pains, especially muscle aches and stiffness.
This requires repeated stretching of the muscles daily (best) or weekly (2-3 times per week). This helps to warm up the muscles and joints and reduce stress on the body.
Joint pain
Joint pain is probably the most common condition people face, and it mainly affects older or overweight people. It often stems from a variety of reasons, including a lack of essential nutrients, weak bones, and inadequate exercise. Some places where people often find pain are the knees, wrists, shoulders, and hips.
The knees and hips are the hardest hit because they are responsible for our balance and mobility.
Practicing yoga can help increase and strengthen the mobility and function of your joints. Some common yoga poses to practice include:

Triangular shapes
This stance is perfect for the entire body, as it reinforces the muscles around the knee, hip, and shoulder joints.
You can utilize a yoga obstruct for help on the off chance that you can't arrive at the ground serenely.
Ensure your back foot is forward and center around fixing your hips while gazing upward. Hold for 10-20 seconds and rehash on the opposite side.
Warrior II works comparable muscles to Triangle yet additionally carries increasingly stretch to your quads.

Headache
Chronic headaches and migraines also plague many people, and this only gets worse as we continue to add more stress and distraction to our lives. Yoga has as many mental benefits as physical benefits. Meditation can do wonders to help you let go of life's many nuances and focus on the things that matter. A significant side effect of this is also the reduction of stress and anxiety.
Practice meditation regularly to ease some of these pains. If you find you need more, try the following:

Sitting forward bend
This posture can help ease some of the tension built up in your head and help you see again. It also works great to increase flexibility in your hamstrings!
Just focus on leaning forward as long as you can comfortably hold the pose, then hold it for 30 seconds. Repeat 3x for optimal effects.
If it is due to natural movements over time or previous injuries, knee movements come not only from the kneecaps and the surrounding muscles and joints but also from the quadriceps muscles.
Take care not to worsen knee pain. Make sure you enter the postures slowly and stop where you feel comfortable. If you feel more pain, ease the stretch.

Back pain
Back pain is the one I hear the most about grumblings, uncommonly low back torment. It torments such countless individuals and can be brought about by a wide range of components, for example, age, weight, and, most importantly, our chiefly inactive way of life. A great many people sit in the vehicle while in transit to work,, sit at a desk to work, sit during meals, and then come home and sit on the couch all night. Sitting can even cause strain on the neck and lower back. Compiled over time, it can cause chronic pain and other problems.

Cobra poses
This posture is delicate on the back, however but can also help strengthen it actively.
It is a pose with which you can choose to work or simply go through the movements actively. Be sure to stretch your back muscles consciously.
Lie on your stomach and place your hands on one foot in front of you, shoulder-width apart. Gently lift with core and back muscles.

MAINTAIN OR IMPROVE THE HEALTH
OF THE JOINTS

Joint torment can make it hard to perform day by day errands or activities. In any case, standard development is essential to keep the joints sound. Yoga, an antiquated practice, maybe the ideal activity to prevent and treat the modern epidemic of joint pain. Soft and low impact, it promotes circulation, strengthens the muscles around the joints, increases flexibility, and improves bone health.

If joint pain comes on suddenly during an activity or develops gradually, it can be debilitating and depressing. 4 But joint pain is usually inevitable, and you can almost always do something to improve it.Pain requires judgment and reflection. Is your pain sharp, which means it lasts for hours or a few days? Is it the result of repeated activity or movement? Provided that this is true, rest and recuperation might be fundamental and accommodating. which means it goes on for a considerable length of time or years, the formula is quite often more significant movement, not rest.

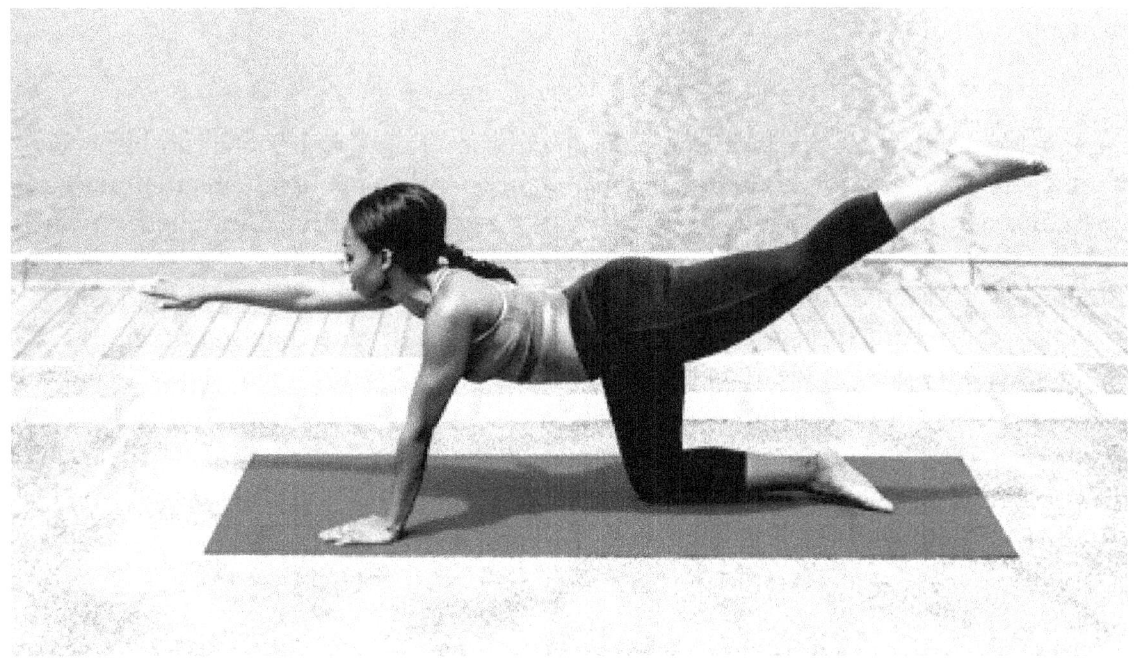

Joint inflammation (a general term used to portray joint agony, firmness, and growing) can be the result of several medical conditions, such as Lyme disease, fibromyalgia, autoimmune disease, or cancer. More than a hundred different types of arthritis cause joint pain, including degenerative, inflammatory, infectious, and metabolic models. Osteoarthritis, a condition in which articular cartilage and bone degenerate, is the most common type of arthritis.

Osteoarthritis generally develops gradually in old age and usually Influences the hands, knees, hips, or spine. Individuals used to trust it was an inescapable piece of maturing or the result of wear and tear from doing too many shocking exercises. Doctors once prescribed rest. However, this paradigm is changing. Today it is increasingly understood that joints need to move regularly to stay healthy, and physical activity almost always improves joint pain, not worse it.

Wear it or lose it
Today, instead of a disease caused by too much exercise, the high prevalence of arthritis can best be explained by the modern sedentary lifestyle. When a person is inactive, the muscles, tendons, and ligaments become weak and unable to support the joints adequately. . Also, regular movement is required to circulate synovial fluid, a smooth substance that nourishes and repairs cartilage around the joints. About 30 percent of the United States populace is inert, and older people are more likely to be physically inactive than younger people. It is probably not a coincidence that older people also experience joint pain more often.

Yoga for the joints
Antiquated profound conventions can be trying to convert into western culture. Yoga generally joins a progression of asanas (physical stances) with contemplation and pranayama (breathing activities). The helpful advantages of yoga can be identified with both unwinding and care and use.
Research confirms the impressive benefits of yoga for joint health. In one study, doing yoga helped osteoarthritis patients reduce pain and stiffness better than standard physical therapy. In another study, yoga three times a week significantly reduced pain. They improved overall health, vitality, and mental health in patients with osteoarthritis of the knee and rheumatoid arthritis, an autoimmune inflammatory disease. In other studies, yoga decreased the torment and expanded capacity in individuals with osteoarthritis of the hands and diminished joint agony in bosom malignant growth survivors.

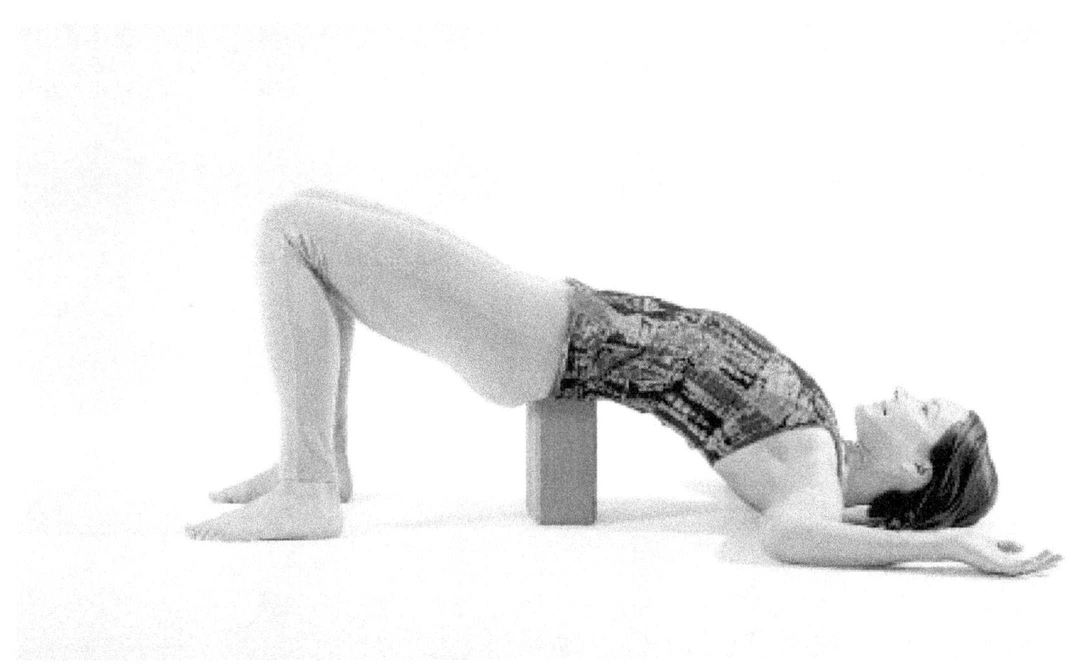

Yoga classes are offered at rec centers, and public venues in the United States, yet not all yoga is made equivalent. On the off chance that you have joint agony, do some exploration, and pick your yoga practice admirably. Yoga wounds are on the ascent, particularly in more seasoned grown-ups. Seventy-four percent of individuals who did yoga saw upgrades in existing agony; however, 21 percent of individuals encountered a worsening of existing torment.

Start where you are

New to yoga and have joint torment, locate a smooth and exact approach to work out. Gentle and casual developments are the ideal approach to help the mending procedure. Abstain from stressing or stressing, which can decline joint torment.

CONCLUSION

Yoga is a subject that can be seen as intellectually and may contain some useful and helpful ideas.

Yoga can be incorporated by adopting specific postures that change the nature of sanskaras.

Yoga can be included by living in an ashram environment while trying to be aware of the physical, mental, and spiritual dimensions.

Yoga can be learned in a classroom as a science, as psychology, as an applied subject, to provide a new understanding and understanding of the life process, in areas where karma is performed, in the regions that form the inner being in terms of consciousness, emotional development, the experience of harmony or balance, which ultimately culminates in the knowledge of samadhi and the fullness of wisdom, prajna.

A state of yoga can be achieved when wisdom is established. This is the vision of the seers who produced the Satyananda yoga. This yoga comes as a way of life, comprehension, and disposition. It is introduced as an essential piece of everyday exercises, of understanding dharma and kartavya, commitments, and obligations, and attempting to consider the to be the world as a gradually creating and creating unit.

These are the components of Satyananda yoga. Many yoga teachers and their schools have developed their yoga brand. Some have followed and spread the path of hatha yoga, some bhakti-yoga, others jnana yoga or kundalini yoga. Still, others have followed different trends in yoga.

Satyananda yoga, also known as Bihar yoga, follows a pattern in yoga, that endeavors to adjust to the conditions of regular day to day existence and, as a significant aspect of life, make an alternate degree of comprehension about wants, edifices, restraints, connections, and interests.

One of the highlights of Satyananda yoga is the practice of yoga as sadhana. To perfect yoga, one must try to develop a tyaga or renunciation. Many applicants feel that they can give up certain things that they may not need, but there is a tendency to become attached to the objects, people, and ideas with which there is an association.
Renunciation should not be isolated from the beauty of life. For those who consider it isolation and try to be what they are not, the tyaga is a complicated process. However, some people go through this process and achieve enlightenment.

When there is a need for self-expression, society offers different areas to meet those needs. Each phase of life has been given different sets of karmas and dharmas, and various roles can be played in these different phases.
In grihastha ashrama or the presence of ahead of the family, one can play the role of a responsible and supportive citizen of society, in which he expresses his needs, achievements, and thoughts and fulfills what one wants to accomplish throughout everyday life.
In brahmacharya ashrama or understudy life, there is the opportunity to learn, comprehend, enter, appreciate, and outfit yourself with the way to prevail throughout everyday life...